The Essiac Report

RICHARD THOMAS

The Essiac Report

*The true story of a Canadian herbal cancer remedy
and of the thousands of lives it continues to save.*

**Published by
The Alternative Treatment
Information Network**

**1244 Ozeta Terrace
Los Angeles
CA 90069
1-310-278-6611**

ISBN 0-9639818-0-3
Manufactured in the United States of America.
Typography and Cover Design by: Fontographics, L.A.

Third Edition.

Publisher's Cataloging in Publication

Thomas, Richard, 1946-

    The Essiac report: the true story of a Canadian herbal cancer
remedy and of the thousands of lives it continues to save / Richard
Thomas. -- 3rd ed.
    p. cm.
    ISBN 0-9639818-0-3

    1. Cancer--Alternative treatment. 2. Herbs--Therapeutic use.
3. Caisse, Rene, ca. 1889-1978.   I. Title.

RC271.A62T46 1994   616'.994069
                                     QBI94-920

TABLE OF CONTENTS

Prologue

"YOU HAVE CANCER," probably the most dreaded diagnosis a patient can ever receive. Just the word CANCER is enough to conjure images of hopeless, unremitting suffering, an unimaginably painful one way trip to the great unknown. A trip forced upon us long before we're ready to embark on our final journey. We'll be leaving our loved ones. We're marked, doomed, forsaken. We're finished. It's CANCER!

A single word is uttered and your life seemingly comes to an end. It's really quite astonishing what one word can do to our perception of reality. But what *is* the reality of cancer? What does the word actually mean? Is it necessarily synonymous with DEATH? Do the collective beliefs held by the "Medical Establishment" concerning cancer and its "proper" treatment serve to empower the patient, or the disease?

If you have any experience at all with traditional medicine you already know that cancer is considered by most medical professionals as a very big deal! A serious condition, indeed. Major. A killer! Thus it follows that such a serious life threatening condition as *cancer* takes an equally serious response, in order to save the afflicted patient. Right? After all, something foreign, evil, unknown has invaded the patient's body and is rapidly mutating, growing, ruthlessly devouring the patient's very existence. In order to stop this insidious killer traditional medical science has developed some rather lethal weapons. Surgery, radiation, and "poison" (chemotherapy), being the first weapons of choice by most oncologists.

But it's a rather curious form of warfare to say the least. Everybody seems to agree that the enemy (cancer) is incredibly powerful, always lurking, and can attack anyone suddenly in many insidious ways. Yet very little is done to prevent the attack. In fact we do quite the opposite, supplying the enemy with endless streams of advanced weaponry: insecticides, carcinogenic chemicals, tobacco and radiation, to name just a few. To make matters infinitely worse, we usually neglect our own defense forces (the immune system) and then we are utterly shocked when the enemy attacks and gets the upper hand. There is very little if any concern about how the enemy was able to invade in the first place. Were the lookouts asleep? Was there no warning of an impending attack? Where are the weak points that allowed the invader to get the upper hand? More importantly, there is almost no attention given to helping the body's already battle-hardened (albeit neglected) standing army, *the immune system*, repel the attacker from within.

In fact, when the counterattack begins, it's mounted with such ferocity *from without* that the body's own defensive forces mistake the intended attack against cancer, as an attack against the entire body... *which in fact it is!* The immune system has no other alternative than to valiantly fight back, weakening it still further.

At the present time the "Medical Establishment" (although they may argue to the contrary) has no proven "smart bombs." When it comes to killing cancer it's usually attempted with something resembling saturation bombing. And we all know what happens to innocent bystanders when you carpet bomb an entire city to kill a handful of guerrillas. *A lot of people die.* Chemotherapy and radiation are for the most part indiscriminate killers. They can definitely kill cancer cells but at what cost? Surgery can be a bit more precise but again at what cost to the "integrity" of the organism?

It is precisely the type of warfare the Medical Establishment has waged that has led some skeptics to conclude that the cure in most cases is no better, and sometimes much worse, than the actual disease. "We are not winning the war," say the critics.

That is not to say there have been no victories... there have. But the war that has been enthusiastically waged against cancer for decades is making very little headway. We may, in fact, be in worse shape than we were on Dec. 23, 1971, when president Nixon signed the National Cancer Act declaring all-out war against cancer. The cure was promised by the Bicentennial. Twenty-three years, billions of dollars and millions of deaths later, no cure is in sight. Are we losing the war? The critics refer to some alarming statistics to make their point. Ralph W. Moss, author of *The Cancer Industry* and Dr. Samuel Epstein, professor of occupational environmental medicine at the University of Illinois, have this to say:

"Cancer now strikes one in three and kills one in four Americans, 500,000 last year alone. Since 1950, overall incidence rates have increased by 40 percent. Cancers of the breast, and of prostate and colon in men, have escalated 60 percent; cancer in children 30 percent. Less common cancers have increased more than 100 percent. Our ability to cure most advance cancers scarcely has improve since 1971. For example, the five year survival rate for non-localized breast cancer remains a static 18 percent.

But what about the emerging 'cures' we were promised, such as taxol or genetic engineering? Remember the cancer vaccine? Remember interferon, miracle cure of the 70's? In truth, few scientists believe their work will result in cures any time soon. But such hype secures next year's funding for hungry bureaucrats and researchers."

To be sure, the generals leading the war against cancer have become a lot richer. Their armies have grown, their arsenals have increased exponentially. Their authority and power to wage war in whatever manner they see fit remains unquestioned. So powerful is the Medical Establishment that they appear to shun anyone who has a novel approach or *new weapon* which might turn the tide, unless it meets their criteria as a "credible" weapon. But their criteria is so steeped in bureaucracy and the costs so prohibitive that only the powerful chemical, pharmaceutical and biotechnology companies are able to play the game.

Some of the most severe critics put forth the notion that the Medical Establishment is involved in a *grand conspiracy* to make mega bucks off millions of unsuspecting cancer victims. It is their firm belief that the Medical Establishment reaps such enormous profits from the treatment of cancer that they have no intention of eventually finding a cure. After all, argue the critics, if a cure were found lucrative research grants would disappear and billions of dollars of revenue generated from surgery and other forms of traditional treatments would simply dry up. They bolster their position by showing the closely interlocking professional and financial interests between the principal components of the Medical Establishment, supposedly leading the war against cancer. Namely, the NCI, the American Cancer Society (ACS), the twenty-odd comprehensive cancer centers, such as New York's Memorial Sloan-Kettering and Boston's Dana-Farber Cancer Institute, the extensive network of NCI and ACS contractees and grantees at most major universities, the leading pharmaceutical houses, and the Food And Drug Administration (FDA), which regulates the marketplace on behalf of the very industries it is supposed to oversee.

Seen in the shadow of huge profits the Medical Establishment does appear to lend credence to those who would argue in favor of a *grand conspiracy* to bilk the public. However, it is more complex than that.

To lump tens of thousands of professionals currently engaged in the research and treatment of cancer into one large group of conniving profit mongers, greedily taking advantage of cancer victims, is unfair. Without a doubt many medical professionals have dedicated their lives to eradicating this devastating disease.

But given their very real dedication and commitment to eradicating cancer and the enormous amount of money spent to advance their commitment, why is there so little progress? *The numbers don't lie.* Could it be that the answer to the cancer riddle lies elsewhere, beyond our venerated research centers, beyond our "top" hospitals, beyond our love affair with modern technology... could it be that the answer has been with us all along, humbly waiting, abundant in the mystery, magic and true curative powers of nature?

———————◆———————

This report is about the dramatic history and development of a very different kind of treatment for cancer, called Essiac. A treatment at once simple, inexpensive, highly effective and natural; a treatment with virtually no side effects and available to anyone. A treatment that has restored health to thousands of cancer victims, most of them pronounced as hopeless by their own physicians.

As you read this report it is important that you not look to the obvious. You will certainly see evidence of what seems like the Medical Establishment's effort to suppress the use of Essiac as a credible cancer treatment. Critics of the Medical Establishment will be inclined to conclude that the history of Essiac is yet more proof of a *grand conspiracy.*

Look deeper and you will see that the story of Essiac is really the story of the perennial conflict between the makers and defenders of what *they* believe is reality and the courageous human beings who hold to a different perspective. It is a story as old as the history of mankind itself. From the trials of Socrates and Galileo, to the Salem witch hunts, and on to the present assault by the FDA against "natural" therapies, anyone who has ever truly challenged the current collective belief system puts themselves in great jeopardy, despite the fact that in many cases history ultimately lands firmly on their side. This conflict will always exist, not because the establishment is inherently evil by nature, but rather because authority, by its very nature, exists solely to defend the status quo. Most people, and especially the authorities, do not like wake-up calls. Destroying illusions is very dangerous.

The people who run the Medical Establishment are no different from other people holding positions of authority. On the one hand they must "protect" society from what they believe is a threat to its well being – in their case, "Quackery." On the other hand they must defend their precious collective belief system, referred to as "Modern Medicine."

Here now is the story of Essiac, the story of an ancient herbal remedy and of the remarkable human beings who have used it to great benefit and thus defied, *and still defy to this day,* cancer's "established" course of events. We hope their victories will be an inspiration to you in your self-evident, open-minded search for the truth.

A word from the Author and The Alternative Treatment Information Network:

Much has already been written about Essiac, some of it confusing and contradictory. Its history in Canada as an incredibly effective natural treatment for cancer has been well reported in numerous magazines and newspapers for the past 65 years. There have been books published, radio and TV programs produced, even a video is being sold which purports to reveal Essiac's original formula and how to prepare it. However, although Essiac may be well known in Canada, very few people in the United States have heard of it.

Has there been a conspiracy of silence, as many people have charged, perpetrated by the American Medical Establishment to keep information about Essiac out of your hands? Maybe, and maybe not. So far our presses haven't been shut down nor have any copies of *The Essiac Report* been confiscated. And we doubt that this will happen. However, after reading this report some of you may disagree.

Is Essiac a cure for cancer? We can say this: All you are about to read is true to the best of our knowledge. We have carefully researched all information available about Essiac... *virtually everything that has ever been printed*. We have conducted numerous interviews with people who have treated themselves with Essiac and claim to have recovered from terminal cancer. We have tried to the best of our ability to separate truth from fiction, fact from fantasy. We have included every possible document which we feel will help present the clearest and most accurate information that exists about Essiac. The information you are about to discover may save your life. Please read this report carefully and thoroughly.

Section One

The Reign Of Saint Rene
1922-1978

In the annals of "natural" cancer remedies Essiac is in a category by itself. The original developer of Essiac, Rene Caisse, in defiance of the authorities, successfully treated thousands of terminal cancer victims for more than 50 years, yet she never charged for her services, and never tried to make a profit from her remarkable discovery. That alone should give rise to serious interest. If you look today at alternative cancer treatments the story is somewhat different. Although the prices for most alternative cancer treatments are less than those charged by traditional medicine, they are steep. Many individuals and organizations who offer alternative cancer therapies are definitely profiting from the disease. Not so with Rene Caisse. Indeed Rene was offered huge sums of money just to divulge the formula, but always she refused. Whether or not her decision was ultimately an intelligent one we'll leave you to decide.

The Discovery

In 1922 Rene Caisse was head nurse at the Sisters of Providence Hospital in Haileybury, Ontario, Canada. She was 33, a Catholic from a typical catholic family of eleven children, bright and extremely dedicated to her profession. One evening while going about her duties she noticed a patient, an elderly woman, who had a strangely scarred breast. Rene felt unusually compelled to ask the woman what had happened. What she was to discover determined the future course of Rene's entire life.

The patient revealed to Rene that more than 20 years earlier she had come from England to join her husband who was working as a prospector in Northern Ontario. Shortly after she arrived a hardened mass appeared on her breast. The area where they were camping was inhabited by Ojibwa Indians and by *luck* they befriended an "old Indian medicine man."

He was made aware of her condition. Not exhibiting the alarm most people have when encountering what surely looked like a serious problem, he offered to help heal her. He had a remedy, he said, which was given to his people by the *grand fathers*, "a holy drink that would purify her body and place it back in balance with the great spirit." She and her husband respected the Indian's kind offer, but being from a culture that considered Indian remedies as little more than superstition, they declined his help. The couple instead decided to journey to Toronto, and there their worst fears were confirmed. Cancer! The breast would have to be removed, immediately.

It hit them hard. The woman had recently lost a friend after a radical mastectomy. Plus they were almost destitute at that time, no money for hospitals or an expensive operation. The woman could not forget the kindness and certainty in the eyes of the old Indian. Modern culture aside, she decided to return and try his remedy. What he gave her was a pleasant tasting herbal tea which she was instructed to drink twice a day until her body was back in "harmony with the great spirit." The medicine man also taught her how to make it on her own.

When Rene encountered the English woman more than twenty years later, her breast was scarred but certainly not cancerous. Rene asked her for the recipe:

> "I was very interested and wrote down the names of the herbs she had used. Knowing that at that time doctors threw up their hands when cancer was discovered in a patient, my thought was that if I should ever develop cancer, I would use it."

Two years later Rene had occasion to use the recipe, but not on herself. Her favorite aunt Mireza had been diagnosed as having terminal cancer of the stomach and liver. Rene was quite familiar with the eventual outcome. She had witnessed firsthand the terrible agony of cancer victims. She was also intimately aware of the advances of modern medical science. Radium therapy, the latest "breakthrough," burned and mangled tissue so badly that most patients experienced an agonizingly painful death after being exposed to this type of therapy.

Rene asked her aunt's physician, Dr. R. O. Fisher, if she might try the old Indian's recipe. Dr. Fisher was skeptical but admitted that at this late stage he had nothing better to offer and consented. She gathered the herbs and brewed the tea.

After two months of daily treatments her aunt got better, a lot better. She lived another twenty years.

Needless to say both Rene and Dr. Fisher were impressed. Rene, who was living with her mother in Toronto, decided, along with the now not so skeptical Dr. Fisher, to try the herbal brew on other patients who had been diagnosed as having "terminal" cancer. When they were treated with the herbal tea, they too showed dramatic improvement. Word spread.

The Early Years

In the 1920's *(as it is today?)* "real" medicine, was thought to be more effective when it was injected. Rene and Dr. Fisher reasoned that if they got such dramatic results with the old Indian remedy by administering it orally they might get even better results if they injected it.

The first person to receive an injection was a man from Lyons, New York, who had cancer of the throat and tongue. With Dr. Fisher's assistance, Rene injected the herbal remedy straight into the man's tongue. The immediate reaction was somewhat unsettling. The patient began to shake uncontrollably, his tongue swelling to the point where it had to be flattened with a spatula to allow him the opportunity to breathe. But after approximately twenty minutes, the swelling and shaking subsided. The patient, who never received another injection, *(and wasn't about to!)* reported that the cancer *did* stop growing, and he was able "to enjoy a pleasant life for some time thereafter."

Rene and Dr. Fisher were encouraged by the results but knew more study should be done on the herbal remedy before they injected their next patient.

They converted Rene's mother's basement on Parkside Drive in Toronto into a laboratory, where she and Dr. Fisher began experiments on mice inoculated with human cancer. In Rene's words:

> "It took Dr. Fisher and I about two years to find out just what ingredients could be given hypodermically without a reaction, and by elimination we found the ingredients that directly reduced the growth of the cancer. However, I found that the other ingredients, which could not be injected, were necessary to the treatment in order to carry off the destroyed tissue and infections thrown off by the malignancy. So by giving the injection to destroy the mass of malignant cells and giving the medicine orally to purify the blood, I was able to get the best results."

It was during this initial perfecting period of the old Indian remedy that the name Essiac was chosen. Essiac is simply Rene's last name, Caisse, in reverse.

The Medical Authorities Were less Than Impressed

Other doctors, hearing about Rene's work from Dr. Fisher, began sending Rene their hopeless cases. An 80 year old man, J. Smith, showed up with a hideous, hemorrhaging malignant growth on his face. Within 24 hours, the bleeding had stopped. After several Essiac treatments the growth began to reduce in size and the large holes in his chin started to heal.

More patients were sent to Rene, by doctors who had pronounced them as hopeless. On the strength of what these doctors saw (many of their former terminal patients made miraculous recoveries after being treated with Essiac) they signed a petition to the Department of National Health and Welfare in

Ottawa, asking that Rene be given facilities to do independent research on a scale worthy of her discovery. Their petition read as follows:

> To whom it may concern:
>
> We, the undersigned, believe that the treatment for cancer given by Nurse R. M. Caisse can do no harm and that it relieves pain, will reduce the enlargement of tumors, and will prolong life in hopeless cases.
>
> To the best of our knowledge, she has not been given a case to treat until everything in medical and surgical science has been tried without effect and even then she was able to show remarkably beneficial results on those cases at that late stage.
>
> We would be interested to see her given an opportunity to prove her work in a large way. To the best of our knowledge she has treated all cases free of any charge and has been carrying on this work over the period of the past two years. Signed:
>
> R. N. Fisher (LRCP, MRCH0)
> R. A Blye (MB)
> E. T. Hoidge (MB, LRCP, MRCP)
> Chas. H. Hair (MDCM)
> S. Moore (MDCM)
> H. T. William (MD)
> J. C. Robert (MB)
> J. A. McInnis (MD)

The Department of Health and Welfare was less than impressed. They promptly sent two investigating doctors empowered with the proper documents to have Rene arrested.

> "When they arrived and found that I was working with nine of the most eminent doctors in Toronto and heard their opinions, they did not arrest me. In fact, one of them (Dr. W. C. Arnold) became so interested that he arranged to have me work on mice at the Christie Street Hospital Laboratories with Dr. Norich and Dr. Locheed. These mice were inoculated with Rous Sarcoma. I kept the mice alive for 52 days, which was longer than anyone else had been able to do."

This was Rene's first experience with the medical authorities. It wouldn't be the last. Previously she couldn't have imagined that anyone would question a treatment for cancer which was completely safe and obviously effective, especially the very doctors who knew just how hard cancer was to heal and who, she was convinced, truly wanted to heal the sick. She was now aware that the medical profession was interested in far more than healing sickness. She had won her first skirmish, but the war was on.

———◆———

By this time Rene was totally committed to her work with cancer patients. When her mother moved back to Bracebridge, Rene rented an apartment on Sherbourne Street in Toronto. She gave up her nursing job and devoted herself full time to her patients. More than *30* a day were now showing up at her doorstep.

The tenants living in her apartment building were not amused. The neighbors were mortified. Too much activity, too many cars on their quiet tree-lined street. They complained! She moved. As it happened, because she charged nothing for her treatments, relying instead on her patients kindly but usually modest donations, she needed to move anyway to a less expensive location. She settled in a modest house in Peterborough, Ontario. One of her first visitors was a policeman armed with a warrant for her arrest:

> "I had just nicely settled in (Peterborough) when a rap came at the door about eight o'clock one morning. There was a man who said he was there to issue a warrant for my arrest for malpractice. I had some letters from the Minister of Health and the College of Physicians and Surgeons saying they would not interfere with me as long as I didn't make a charge, so I wasn't expecting anything like this. However, I excused myself to go upstairs and get dressed, and in the meantime the man sat down to read the letter and papers, and when I came down he said he was not going to arrest me, but was going back to talk to his boss, Dr. R. T. Noble, the registrar of the College of Physicians and Surgeons.
>
> I was frantic. I thought this would probably happen again, so I called and made an appointment with the Minister of Health, Dr. J. M. Robb. Some of the patients and doctors I'd worked with came with me, and Dr. Robb told me I wouldn't be interfered with again as long as I didn't make a charge for my treatments, and had a written diagnosis of cancer from a doctor for each patient."

Note that the emphasis was that she not charge for treating people. *That privilege we presume was reserved for only those medical professionals who had demonstrated a more accepted and effective form of treatment?*

A Clinic Is Born

News of Rene's successes continued to spread. The first major newspaper article, entitled, "Bracebridge Girl Makes Notable Discovery Against Cancer," appeared in 1932 in the Toronto Star. Rene was becoming famous. And as such, the authorities would eventually have to take stronger action.

After the article appeared Rene was overwhelmed with requests for help. She also received several business proposals. A Toronto businessman, Ernest H. Ashley, went so far as to have a contract prepared which offered Rene her own clinic, $20,000 within the first year of signing, an additional $2,000 annual salary, and $100,000 operating capital and stock in a corporation to be formed. All that was required of her was to "assign and set over all her right, title and interest in the said formula, above referred to."

These were big bucks in 1932, she turned them down. As we'll further discover, profit was never a consideration with Rene. Her interest was in saving lives; she never wavered.

Rene continued to treat and cure more and more patients. On June 17, 1933, she received a letter from the Deputy Minister of Hospitals for Ontario. He wrote that he had heard only positive reports about her treatment and was therefore highly interested in finding out more details.

About the same time, Dr. A. F. Bastedo of Bracebridge Ontario, let Rene treat one of his patients who had terminal bowel cancer. When the patient recovered, Dr. Bastedo was so impressed he convinced the Town Council of Bracebridge to make the British Lion Hotel, repossessed for back taxes, available to Rene for a cancer clinic. As Rene tells it:

> "The Mayor and Council were very enthusiastic and with their aid and the aid of friends, relatives, and patients, I furnished an office, dispensary, reception room and five treatment rooms. Here I worked for almost eight years with a large 'CANCER CLINIC' sign on the door."

Rene opened her clinic in 1934 and almost immediately it became a bustling, thriving center of hope for the hopeless, a veritable last chance oasis.

Homemaker's, a Canadian national magazine, described the scene:

> Dominion Street took on an atmosphere reminiscent of the famous Shrine of Lourdes, as hopeful pilgrims sought a new lease on life. Cars were parked solidly along its shoulder. People from all walks of life waited patiently to enter the red brick building. Some were carried.
> Others were pushed gently up the steps, while the rest managed on their own. Occasionally, an ambulance would shriek it's arrival as it double-parked. Rene would be seen coming quickly down to it to treat a stretcher case. Always with a doctor standing by, she injected scores of patients every day.

No sooner had the clinic opened than Rene was faced with her most personal bout with cancer. Her mother, 72, was diagnosed with inoperable liver cancer. Rene sought the opinion of Ontario's top specialist, Dr. Roscoe Graham who informed Rene that her mother's liver was, "a nodular mass. It's only a matter of days." Rene didn't tell her mother she had cancer, instead she gave her daily injections of Essiac, explaining to her mother that the medicine was a revitalizing tonic prescribed by her doctor. Rene tells it this way:

> "To make a long story short my mother completely recovered. She passed away quietly after her 90th birthday, without pain, just a tired heart. This repaid me for all of the work, giving my mother 18 years of life she would not have had without Essiac. It made up for a great deal of the persecution I have endured at the hands of the medical people."

As Rene continued to treat cancer victims at her clinic she enjoyed such success that her supporters circulated a petition demanding that the

Department of Health and Welfare support Rene's work. After gathering thousands of signatures the petition was duly presented to Dr. J. A. Faulkner, provincial Minister of Health.

Another petition was presented signed by nine medical doctors:

Wm H. Oaks (Rosseau); M. S. Wittick (Burks Falls); W. Dillane (Powassan); E. J. Ellis (Bracebridge); F. Shannon (Churchill); B.l. Guyatt (Toronto); J. M. Greig (Bracebridge); R. O. Fisher (Toronto); and J. A. McInnis (Timmins).

The doctors, who obviously believed in the importance of Essiac, strongly urged that immediate action be taken to make Essiac available for all cancer sufferers, and that it be kept a Canadian discovery.

Upon receiving this petition, Dr. Faulkner immediately conferred with Sir Frederick Banting, MD, one of the most prestigious physicians in the world, publically credited as the co-discoverer of insulin. Dr. Banting was very interested in what he heard. He already knew of Essiac as early as 1925, when he was made aware of a diabetic woman who had been treated with Essiac for advanced cancer of the bowel. The woman was advised by her doctor, J. A. McInnis, not to use insulin while being treated with Essiac because he thought it might interfere with the effectiveness of Essiac. *(It would not have.)*

After recovering from cancer the woman no longer needed insulin. Her diabetic condition had completely disappeared! When Dr. Banting was told of the case and later investigated it, he concluded that Essiac had somehow "stimulated the pancreas to function normally, thereby healing the diabetes."

Why Dr. Banting did nothing (after learning that Essiac not only healed cancer but apparently diabetes as well) is not known.

However this time, more than ten years later, he did do something. He further investigated the claims made about Essiac, and was so impressed that he invited Rene to actually come to his facility, the Banting Institute in Toronto, to work under his supervision. Dr. Banting's interest in Essiac was seen by Rene's supporters as a major breakthrough. According to Rene, Dr. Banting told her:

"Miss Caisse, I will not say you have a cure for cancer, but you have more evidence of a beneficial treatment for cancer than anyone in the world."

All testing of Essiac at the Banting Institute was to be performed on animals before Rene would be allowed to treat humans. In effect, it meant giving up her work saving human lives at her clinic, while she tried to prove to the "scientific community" the merit of Essiac on lab animals.

Rene felt she had already done her work with mice! Furthermore, when her patients heard that she might be leaving to do research in Toronto, they were terrified – "How could she abandon them?" – while most of the doctors that knew of Dr. Banting's offer strongly urged Rene to take advantage of this "incredible" opportunity to legitimize Essiac.

Rene refused Dr. Banting's offer. Her rationale was simple: too many people would die while she was trying to prove to the Medical Establishment that Essiac saved lives. Most of the doctors that had worked with her were astonished that she would let this opportunity pass. They failed, as they would in the future, to perceive that Rene's primary mission in life was to save human lives *now*. She had something that did just that, and in her mind she didn't need to prove it any further. Her decision came straight from her heart – possibly naive, but certainly praiseworthy.

On Aug 11, 1936, Dr. Banting wrote this to Rene:

"I think you will regret that you have not availed yourself of the offer made by this laboratory. However, if at some future time you again decide to have the treatment investigated, I am sure that Dr. Faulkner and myself would reconsider the matter."
(See Appendix/ Exhibit 1, Page 101.)

Among the lives that Rene stayed in Bracebridge to save was that of Tony Baziuk, a CNR engine watchman who developed lip cancer and was given radium treatments by Dr. McNeill in London, Ontario. His lip was so swollen after the radium treatments he could look at it over the end of his nose. The pain was excruciating. He had to leave his job.

His fellow workers collected enough money to pay his way to Bracebridge from his home in Capreol. He arrived with a written diagnosis from Dr. McNeill stating that he had cancer of the lip, which was more than obvious!

Rene later commented:

"His face was so disfigured, it was unbearable to look at."

One injection of Essiac and Tony felt immediate relief. In only six months he was back on the job, where, in his words, he could:

"Eat for one man, work for three and (when he went home) sleep like a little baby."

He lived another 40 years.

In 1977 May Henderson remembered her journey to Bracebridge in 1937 as follows:

"We liked to get an early start because the clinic was always filled. We tried to get our treatments before lunch, have a bite to eat in Bracebridge, and then drive back. It only took a minute to get the injection and drink the tea, and the patients used to exchange progress report while we waited."

When May went to Rene she had tumors in both breasts, and had been advised by her doctor to have a double mastectomy. She was also to discover on a subsequent visit to her doctor that she had a tumor the size of a grapefruit in her uterus. She was almost too weak to move, but she had a horror of surgery and would have nothing of it.

"My color was a muddy yellow, my hair thin and lifeless and my eyes, ordinarily blue, were gray and stony, I hemorrhaged so badly I thought I would die, and couldn't stand up for any length of time"

May's physician, Dr. J. A. McInnis, concluded that she was hopeless and sent her to Rene. She began the Essiac injections. In three months May was back at work. She tells of her recovery this way:

"At first, the lumps seemed to grow harder, but then the turning point came and I discharged great masses of fleshy material."

Still healthy in 1977 when she recalled her experiences, she never had a recurrence.

Are these cases simply anecdotal, as the medical establishment would have us believe, or do they reveal a treatment that was truly remarkable?

Another case, which Rene felt was typical of the recoveries made while she was treating patients at her clinic, was Nellie McVittie who when she told her story to *Homemakers* in 1977 was very much alive and healthy.

When Nellie arrived at Rene's clinic in 1935 she was carried in, weighing a mere 86 pounds and badly hemorrhaging. Her doctor in Sudbury, Dr. Dale, believed she had cancer of the uterus and neck of the womb. The neck of the womb had been cauterized, then further subjected to radium treatments. When Nellie later appeared at the Cancer Commission hearing in 1939, she had this to say:

"Miss Caisse's treatments certainly put me on my feet. I could barely get around at all when I went to her. I weigh about 107 pounds now."

There was really only one incident in the entire eight years in which Rene ran her cancer clinic that, as Rene put it, "marred the serenity of my work and I will never forget it."

Apparently a patient, Mrs. Gilrouth, who was already suffering from an acute embolism, insisted that she come to Rene's clinic for treatment. Her doctor had previously contacted Rene and told her of her condition and that she had an ulcer which would not heal. He asked to please see if the Essiac treatment might help. When Rene injected her with Essiac the patient immediately lost consciousness and died.

According to Rene:

"There were two doctors there but she was dead before they could do anything. I remembered that her doctor had told me that this could happen anytime from an embolism. Her two sons, who were with her, told me that their doctor had warned them that this could happen anytime. They said that she had had a weak spell that morning and they did not want to bring her for treatment, but she had insisted on coming."

The Department of Health and Welfare was notified. They promptly made the press aware of what had happened:

"WOMAN DIES AFTER TREATMENT AT CAISSE CANCER CLINIC"
(Appeared in headlines across Canada.)

Two chief pathologists, Dr. Robinson and Dr. Frankis, were dispatched from Toronto to do an autopsy. An inquest was convened. Rene was later to recall:

> "They did not arrest me but held a 'court' and gave me a 'trial by jury' of twelve men."

The judge was Dr. Smirlie Lawson of Toronto. It was alleged that Rene did not have a written diagnosis from her doctor. It was in fact mislaid, but found in time to present it before appearing in court. The pathologists assured the jury that the patient would have died whether or not she had the Essiac treatment. Their report read as follow:

> Death occurred as a result of an embolism in the pulmonary artery: a condition brought about by a varicose condition. Pulmonary embolism had been evident for years.

Rene was completely exonerated from all blame. Her clinic was not closed and the publicity surrounding the inquest brought even more patients. Sometimes Rene and her volunteer staff, which included doctors and other medical personnel who believed in Rene's work, treated over a hundred patients a day. She was working incredibly long hours, but never once complained. For Rene it was not work. It was a mission of love. All part of God's plan.

Fame, Fortune and Matters of the Heart

By the end of 1937 more petitions were circulated. This time 17,000 signatures were obtained! The government was being forced to act. They would soon either have to shut her down, or sanction her cancer treatment.

At the same time word had spread to the United States. It didn't take long before a group of U.S. businessmen made Rene an offer *they* thought impossible for her to refuse.

Through their attorney they offered Rene the following:

> It is proposed to organize a Foundation (headed by Miss Caisse) which will bear the name of Essiac or Miss Caisse; to make $1 million available for building and equipment; to pay her $50,000.00 a year in addition to royalties from the commercialization of Essiac; to make her a gift of $200,000.00.

Rene was dubious. She felt they would eventually exploit Essiac for profit. She flatly refused their offer.

Think about it for a moment. This was an incredible amount of money she was turning down. Multiply the figures by at least ten to put the amount in today's terms!

Meanwhile a leading diagnostician in Chicago, Dr. Clifford Barbourka, introduced Rene to Dr. John Wolfer who at that time was head of the medical division of Northwestern University. Dr. Wolfer had heard of Rene's work and asked her if she would be interested in treating 30 volunteer patients in various stages of terminal cancer. She would be supervised by five doctors. This time, because she was being asked to treat humans rather than mice, and because there was no stipulation that she hand over her formula, she accepted the offer.

When the news appeared in Canada that Rene would be going to the United States to do further research with Essiac on "real" patients, Premier Hepburn and the Minister of Health were deluged with outraged letters. Angry editorials in newspapers appeared throughout Ontario. "Why was she taking her treatment to the U.S. and abandoning Canada?" "Why was she forced to do her research in the U.S.?"

At this point in Rene's career she knew how to handle the press. She assured her terrified patients and the public, through the press, that she would not abandon Canada. She would only go to Chicago every other week, and would continue her work at home the rest of the time.

She made her trips to Chicago for a year and a half, carrying with her the proper papers endorsed by Dr. Wolfer, which allowed her to clear customs with her medication. She insisted on preparing her own ampules, usually done at night, sometimes very late at night, boiling and steeping the herbs, straining and then bottling them for the next day.

Her schedule was gruelling. She treated her patients in Bracebridge on the weekends, traveled to the King Edward Hotel in Toronto and treated more patients, and then on to Chicago, occasionally falling ill from fatigue and quickly recovering to continue her work. She had no life of her own.

The Chicago doctors were impressed with what they saw. They concluded that Essiac did indeed prolong life, break down tumors, and relieve pain. Dr. Barbourka offered Rene facilities at Chicago's Passavant Hospital if she would move there permanently. Rene refused. In her words:

"I wanted my work recognized in Canada, and I didn't want to abandon my Bracebridge patients."

Again the doctors failed to understand how dedicated Rene was to her patients. The doctors were shocked at her refusal to work permanently in a "real" cancer treatment facility! She returned to her clinic in Bracebridge to devote all of her time to her Canadian patients.

An Avalanche of Support; Skeptics Converted

During the years leading up to 1938 and her legislative battle, records show an ever increasing outcry from the public to have Essiac officially recognized as a "legitimate" cancer treatment. Premier Mitchell Hepburn and the Department of Health were inundated with letters praising Rene and insisting that Essiac be officially sanctioned. Virtually all of the letters received were supportive in the extreme.

Here's just one example that appeared in the Bracebridge Gazette in 1936, written by Mrs. Lehman:

> "I wonder if you people know what a wonderful thing life is – or do you, in your everyday hurry, forget? I had been given three months to live before I came to Miss Caisse. The time is past, and I have received wonderful results. I feel I must do my utmost to bring knowledge to other sufferers of the dread disease, and Miss Caisse has proof she can show (with picture) of what she has done for me, and is doing. Now, people of Bracebridge, give your fellow townswoman your whole-hearted support. Help her in every way necessary, and put Bracebridge on the map as the place with the most wonderful cancer clinic."

Doctors from both the U.S. and Canada, many of them skeptical, would show up at her clinic to observe her work, talk to patients, examine her records, and try to decide for themselves what was happening in Bracebridge.

Dr. Benjamin Leslie Guyatt, MD, who was the curator of the University of Toronto's anatomy department, was a frequent visitor. Here is an excerpt from what he wrote about the clinic:

> "In most cases, distorted countenances became normal, and the pain reduced as treatment proceeded. The relief from pain is a notable feature, as pain in these cases is very difficult to control. On checking authentic cancer cases, it was found that hemorrhage was rapidly brought under control in many difficult cases; open lesions of lip and breast responded to treatment; cancer of the cervix, rectum and bladder have been caused to disappear; and patients with cancer of the stomach diagnosed by reputable physicians and surgeons have returned to normal activity.
>
> I do know that I have witnessed in this clinic a treatment which brings about restoration through destroying the tumor tissues and supplying that something which improves the mental outlook on life and facilitates re-establishment of physiological function."

One of the most skeptical doctors to investigate Rene's treatments was Dr. Richard Leonardo, coroner of Rochester, New York. He was a cancer specialist who had written numerous books on the subject and had travelled extensively to observe advanced surgical procedures. Rene recalled his visit to her clinic this way:

> "He was a big bluff fellow, and he was very skeptical and plain-spoken. He said he didn't believe I had any remedy, but after he talked to

the patients he said you're doing them good, but it's your personality and the hope you offer them! He took his time talking to patients and other doctors. Then just before he left, he sat down on my couch and hammered on the side of it and said: 'Well, by God, you've got it! But the medical profession isn't going to let you do this to me. I spent seven years in medical school, and I've written books.'

He told me that if my treatment of a simple hypodermic injection was accepted, he'd have to go home and tear up his books and discard his surgical instruments. I was pleased that he was impressed, because when he came he was so skeptical."

Dr. Emma Carson arrived from California. She had originally decided to stay at Rene's clinic for only one day. She left 24 days later. Here's an excerpt of what she discovered:

"I firmly resolved that my investigation be based on unprejudiced judgement. The vast majority of Miss Caisse's patients were brought to her after surgery, radium, ghvbs, emplastrums, etc. had failed to be helpful and the patients were pronounced incurable or hopeless cases. The progress obtainable and the actual results from Essiac treatments, and the rapidity of repair were absolutely marvelous, and must be seen to be believed. My skepticism neither yielded nor became subdued by the hopes and faith so definitely expressed by the patients and their friends.

As I reviewed, compared and summarized my data, records, case histories, etc. I realized that skepticism had deserted me. When I arrived I contemplated remaining 12 hours: I remained 24 days. I examined results obtained on 400 patients."

Could all of what these doctors observed be simply anecdotal?

The Battle To Legalize Essiac

By 1938 Rene's support had grown enormously. Another petition was circulated. This time it garnered 55,000 signatures! The public along with many doctors and professionals from all walks of life were demanding in no uncertain terms that Rene be allowed to, in effect, practice medicine without a license.

Frank Kelly, a member of the legislature, went so far as to have election handbills printed that displayed Rene's picture and quoted her as saying she had Premier Hepburn's assurance that legislation would soon be introduced which would allow her to operate her clinic legally.

Imagine if you will the wrath Rene was about to incur from a Medical Establishment firmly entrenched in their faith in the wonders of modern medicine. A Medical Establishment that legally held the power to crush anyone who had the audacity to practice the art of healing not in accordance with the precepts of the ordained faith.

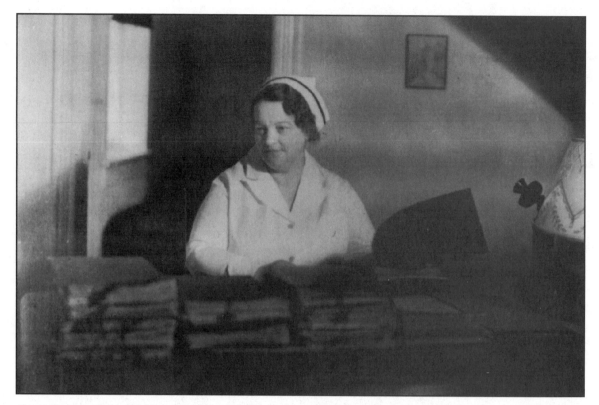

Rene Caisse sitting in March 1938 with her piles of 55,000 names. Many M.D.'s signed this petition which accompanied the Private member Bill to the floor of the Ontario Legislature to permit Rene Caisse R.N. to practice medicine without a license and continue treating cancer patients openly.

In March, 1938, a private bill was introduced by Frank Kelly which proposed that Rene Caisse be officially authorized to "practice medicine in Ontario in the treatment of cancer in all its forms and of human ailments and condition resulting therefrom."

Rene desperately wanted legislation passed allowing her to treat patients before they were diagnosed as terminal, because the doctors were not sending her patients until the last stages of the disease, patients who had already been subjected to the traumas of traditional cancer treatments. They were all but killing her patients before she was given a chance to help them. In Rene's words:

> "Medical science has nothing to offer the cancer sufferer but X-ray, radium and surgery. Radiation has the opposite effect, it causes cancer. Radium drives it in instead of out and burns the surrounding tissue."

The Medical Establishment naturally perceived the proposed legislation as a direct attack on their credibility, indeed their entire reason for existing. Their response was not surprising.

Dr. Faulkner, who had in the past been sympathetic to Rene, was replaced as Minister of Health by Harold Kirby. Harold "would not see the honor of modern medical science tainted!" In the beginning of March, 1938, the "Kirby Bill" was introduced in the legislature.

Briefly stated, the Kirby Bill was created, according to its defenders, as a way "to get to the truth" about "unorthodox" cancer treatments. Rene's treatment being of course the main target. The Kirby Bill would protect the public because it would discover if "controversial" treatments had merit. The Kirby Bill would therefore have the power to establish a Royal Cancer Commission to investigate all possible cancer treatments.

Rene would be allowed to offer evidence to the Royal Cancer Commission, which would be composed of respected members of the Canadian College of Physicians and Surgeons. If, and only if, her evidence was conclusive, the Cancer Commission would then legalize Essiac. There were however a few minor stipulations:

The formulas for all treatments investigated must be turned over to the Cancer Commission. If one refused to divulge the formula one was subject to a fine of $100 to $500 the first time they were caught treating a patient, and $500 to $2,500 the second time, and for each subsequent offense. Failure to pay the fine could result in 30 days to six months in prison.

But according to the Kirby Bill, all members of the Cancer Commission would be required to maintain the confidentiality of the formulas submitted for review. But if the esteemed members "accidently" or otherwise broke this confidentiality there were of course no penalties for their breach of fiduciary duty.

Rene was outraged when she heard about the bill. She believed if she turned over her formula to the Cancer Commission, they would never keep it secret!

> "The people of Ontario will be paying a group of men to develop something that was developed and discovered 15 years ago. I have developed and proven a cure right here in Bracebridge and I am running a clinic where hundreds of cancer sufferers are being treated and helped. Why then should I be asked to give my formula over to a group of doctors who never did anything to earn it? If the Ontario legislature can pass a law to put me in jail for six months for helping suffering people, I will close my clinic and go to the United States. I shall not buck such opposition."

Naturally Rene's supporters were determined to see that her bill be passed and the Kirby bill defeated. Rene's bill was the first to be debated in the legislature.

According to transcripts, the debate was fierce. Rene's lawyer opened with:

> "Patients and their relatives are reporting that doctors are refusing to give Rene diagnoses of cancer, and that a cabal has been organized by the medical profession against her."

The charge was met with cries of "untrue" and "shame" by members of the legislature.

Another gentleman rose to his feet and declared:

> "My mother was a cancer patient, yet three doctors refused to give her a written diagnosis for Miss Caisse, though they gave it to my mother verbally."

Scores of patients in the gallery applauded his statement with such enthusiasm that Speaker David Croll threatened to expel them from the House, "if you don't settle down!" The speaker went on to say:

> "The Government is setting up a board to deal with these reported cures," (referring to the Cancer Commission to be established when the Kirby bill passed). *A foregone conclusion.*

Members of Parliament, Duckworth, Armstrong and Summerville, all gave impassioned speeches as to why the bill should be passed. Each time they gave the name of a terminal patient they had known personally who had been cured, the gallery erupted in cheers.

One by one patients were allowed to tell of their miraculous turnarounds because of their treatment with Essiac.

And then Rene was allowed to take the stand. The legislature was silent as she spoke:

> "The fact that I can get any results at all should be accepted as a good thing. When I had success, I thought the doctors would welcome me with open arms. I didn't anticipate antagonism from the profession. I expected cooperation and I have every respect for the profession."

She told the legislature she would "gladly" give her formula to the world without any thought of gain:

> "If I knew that it would be given to humanity in the same way. I have never asked a patient for one cent. I have been glad to have donations of one or two dollars but I have never asked a patient if they had money. I treated them whether they had it or not."

All she really wanted was for the medical profession to admit that Essiac had merit, based on the results she had already obtained. Then she would welcome any type of investigation.

> "My clinic is wide open to any investigation at all times."

One is struck at her naivete and bravery. All she wanted was the Medical Establishment to abandon every sacred belief they clung to about the treatment of cancer!

When she finished speaking, a motion was put forth calling for "the bill not to be reported." A vote was taken by a show of hands. Rene's bill was defeated by just *three* votes on the grounds that to allow it would be the same as endorsing her treatment as a *cure* or *effective* remedy. Clearly she had a tremendous amount of support, but in the end it wasn't enough.

A few days later the Kirby bill was easily passed into law. Rene notified her patients that she would be closing her clinic:

"I regret with all my heart closing my cancer clinic here at Bracebridge. I have battled with the medical profession but when it comes to fighting the law of the province it is too much for me."

The Huntsville *Forester* described the scene at Rene's clinic when she told her patients of her decision to close:

Tears began to flow down the cheeks of dozens of cancer victims who had been receiving benefit from their treatment with Miss Caisse, and whose last hope apparently vanished with the announcement of the closing of the clinic. One patient is reported to have fainted, while others, in complete dejection, had to be assisted to their motor cars. Miss Caisse herself was so overcome that she had to leave the scene.

The Premier and the Minister of Health were deluged with letters demanding to know why Rene had been forced to close her doors.

One letter typical of that time was written by Mr. M. M. Andercheck of Timmons, Ontario:

"It has been a very severe blow to me as well as to many of the sufferers to hear that Miss Caisse was forced to close her clinic. I think it is a great injustice to the hundreds of sufferers from the dreadful disease whom Miss Caisse has so greatly benefited.

My wife was one of her patients for the last three months and has gained in health and confidence and was looking forward to regaining her health again. She is only 34 years of age and a mother of a three year old child. It seems such a pity to take away the opportunity from a person her age to regain health and happiness, to which every person is entitled. And leave nothing but despair."

Under incredible public pressure, Premier Hepburn and Health Minister Kirby thought it politically wise to ask Rene to re-open her clinic. She was reassured that she would not be charged under the new Kirby law. She consented. Her patients were overjoyed.

※ ◆ ※

In August, 1938, six physicians with "expertise" in the treatment of cancer were named as members of the newly formed Royal Cancer Commission. They were:

W. C. Wallace, MA, DSc, PhD, LLD, FGS, FRSC, Kingston; R. E. Valin, MD, DS, CM, FRCS, Ottawa; E. A. Collins, BSc, Copper Cliff; W. J. Deadman, BA, MB, Hamilton; T. H. Callahan, MB, Toronto; and G. S. Young, MB, FRCP, Toronto.

Dr. W.C. Wallace and Dr. T. H. Callahan were promptly sent to Bracebridge to interview Rene's patients. Rene was delighted at the prospect. She had nothing to hide, and as she had stated in the legislature, "her clinic was wide open for anyone to investigate." To a person every one of the doctors interviewed gave glowing reports of their treatment with Essiac, *but it didn't really matter.* The purpose of the interviews was little more than a formality, an insignificant prelude to the main event.

Early in March, 1939, public hearings got under way at the Royal York Hotel in Toronto, before the full Cancer Commission. Rene rented one of the hotel ballrooms to accommodate the 387 patients who accompanied her in support. For reasons never fully explained, the Royal Commission allowed just 49 to testify.

The testimony found in the court transcripts of those patients allowed to speak on Rene's behalf gives a vivid picture of what happened during the inquisition. All of Rene's patients who were allowed to testify were absolutely convinced that Essiac had helped them recover from cancer. Some of them told of partial recoveries, others of miraculous recoveries after they had been given up as hopeless by the Medical Establishment.

George Mahon testified:

> "She helped me. If it was not for her, I would be buried."

Elizabeth Stewart testified:

> "After treatment by Nurse Caisse, I'm working every day. I milk five cows, night and morning. I'm right off the farm and have boarders and all in the house, and I have to do it all myself. I owe my life to Miss Caisse and I hope you will do something for her."

Annie Bonar, who had been diagnosed by biopsy at St. Michael's by Dr. E. R. Shannon who said she had cancer of the uterus and bowel, testified:

> "My cancer had spread after radium treatments until my arm had swelled to double its size, and turned black. I went down from 150 pounds to 90 pounds, and then entered St. Michael's to have my arm amputated, but changed my mind on the eve of the operation and went to Bracebridge instead. After four months on the Essiac treatment my arm has returned to normal, and I have gained 60 pounds."

John Thronbury testified that his wife had been diagnosed by X-rays two years previously as having probable cancer of the stomach.

> "She was so weak then that at 72 pounds she had to be carried into the Bracebridge clinic." Mrs. Thronbury testified herself to the royal commission that "I now weigh 107 pounds and can do all of my work." (She lived to be 91 and died in 1975.)

The other patients allowed to testify gave similar reports of dramatic recoveries. *None of it mattered.* The commissioners simply dismissed most of what they heard as improper original diagnoses. Some doctors even denied their own previous diagnoses in letters sent to Dr. R. T. Noble, Registrar of the College of Physicians and Surgeons.

When their recantations were presented in court as evidence against Essiac's effectiveness, Rene's lawyer exploded. Implying that there had to have been pressure applied for the doctors to abandoned their earlier findings, he said:

> "If this matter (of diagnosing) is done so sloppily, there should probably be a commission to investigate that!"

Rene would later state:

> "In the 49 cases examined by the Ontario Cancer Commission, the majority of these had more than the diagnosis of one doctor; some of them had three or four doctors and were told they had cancer and were treated for malignancy before coming to me for Essiac treatment."

During the hearing, several patients described the horror of radium burns and surgery. Almost all of them had been pronounced as terminal. Many sought Rene only after suffering a recurrence following radium or surgery.

Dr. Guyatt, the anatomist from the University of Toronto, was finally allowed to testify:

> "I am satisfied that the patients I saw at Bracebridge were definitely receiving benefit. I would not say (it was) a cure, because a cure of cancer means 25 years. But certainly there has been a great benefit in those cases."

He then went on to describe his considerable experience in diagnosing cancer and stated that the cases he observed had been diagnosed properly.

Nearing the close of the hearing, the chairman declared:

> "What she (Nurse Caisse) is asking us to do is pass on the case histories she had given us, without the Board having any knowledge of what the substance contains, or the theory of its operation or administration."

"Exactly!" responded Rene's lawyer.

After a rather lengthy heated debate between Rene's lawyer and the Commissioners about her refusal to turn over her formula, Commissioner Valin said:

> "You are seriously, I think, prejudicial to your cause in not revealing the formula. We may be favorably impressed. We don't know. As far as we have gone, we cannot tell. There may be something in it, as Dr. Guyatt says. He thinks it is something which should be investigated further. That is what he suggested, to have some independent investigator go ahead, and he appeals to the Ontario Medical Society to have it investigated. That is his impression, and he is a disinterested party. He is not biased. We feel we should like to pursue our observations further, and that is the reason why we want the formula."

With that the inquisition was over for the time being. Two weeks later came the testimony from doctors opposing Rene. *This testimony mattered a great deal.* It possessed the vehemence and zeal worthy of the Medical Establishment's concerted effort to "find out the truth."

Rene listened patiently as Dr. Richards and Dr. Nobel tried to tear her treatment apart. "Many patients had not benefited at all from Essiac," they insisted, "and some had even died!" (*Imagine that; Essiac couldn't cure everybody?*)

Rene responded in kind:

> "A great number of these cases are hopeless cases, who came to me perhaps for treatment, and I tell the family (I did not tell the patient) but I tell the family that it is hopeless, and I cannot hope to do anything other than possibly give them comfort. If they care to take a few treatments they do so, and if they go away and die, then these records go against me."

Commissioner Valin challenged:

> "Apparently you say you cannot cure an advanced case."

Rene snapped back:

> "No, I did not say that. If the organs are destroyed, yes. I cannot build new bodies."

Some of the reports submitted by opposing physicians actually admitted that their former patients claimed to have received benefit from Essiac, at least in the area of pain reduction. In fact, almost all of the hostile reports submitted mentioned Essiac's ability to reduce pain. But these were post mortem reports, and Essiac's ability to reduce pain was only mentioned briefly. Pain relief was not the issue. The issue was to crush Rene.

Finally a tired and weary Rene said to the Commissioners:

> "Dr. Noble and Dr. Richards are both bringing up a lot of patients whom I took on for pity's sake. They are not taking up my proven cases, which have benefited. A great number of these patients came for one or two treatments, and never came back, and I could not save them. I did not want to take them at all, because I knew the cases were hopeless. Every case was given up by the medical profession before I even took it."

The commission was ready to play their trump card. They knew if they asked Rene for her formula she would refuse. Her refusal would be prima fascia evidence that Essiac had no real merit. After all, why else would she refuse to allow her discovery to be analyzed by the "proper authorities?" Surely it would be exposed as a hoax when seen in the divine light of modern medical science!

They asked Rene if she would submit her formula. Once again, she told them she would not turn over the formula because she believed it would be immediately shelved as worthless: In her words:

> "I want to know that suffering humanity will benefit by it. When I can be given that assurance, I am willing to disclose my formula, but I have got to know that it is going to get to suffering humanity."

Chairman Gillanders said he wouldn't admit to any merit before receiving the formula. No one would budge.

In December, 1939, the Commission delivered its Interim Report to Parliament. It stated that in cases where diagnosis had been by biopsy there was only one recovery with Essiac, and two improvements. In cases diagnosed by X-ray, one recovery was attributed to Essiac, and two improvements. In clinically diagnosed cases, two recoveries were attributed to Essiac, and four improvements were noted. The Commission felt there were at least three wrong diagnoses, up to ten questionable ones, and four that were not conclusive. Only eleven were accepted. Out of the eleven, five cures were attributed to previous radium treatments. One of them was Mrs. Annie Bonar, who had been faced with amputation of her arm after a year of radium and X-ray treatments. She had recovered, and it certainly couldn't have been from a simple tea made from plants! It was the radium that delivered Mrs. Bonar, the commission concluded.

Rene had this to say:

> "It is my opinion that the hearing of my case before the Cancer Commission was one of the greatest farces ever perpetrated in the history of man. Over 380 patients came to be heard and the Commission limited the hearing to 49 patients. Then in their report they stated that I had only taken 49 patients to be heard, that X-ray reports were not acceptable as a diagnosis, and that the 49 doctors had made wrong or mistaken diagnoses. It is a sad state of affairs if doctors can diagnose an affliction as 'cancer' and send the patients home with a few months (at most) to live, if they are not sure."

The Cancer Commission in effect had stated that Essiac had no merit and unless she turned over the formula she would be subject to prosecution under the Kirby law.

The Silent Years

Rene kept her clinic open in spite of the Cancer Commissions ruling, but her patients found it more difficult and sometimes impossible to provide Rene with a written diagnosis. Rene became increasingly worried that it was only a matter of time before she would be prosecuted and imprisoned under the Kirby Bill. She closed her clinic in 1942. Her friends described her at that time as "bordering on a nervous breakdown."

For the time being she had taken her fight as far as any one person could against the awesome power and limitless resources of the Medical Establishment.

She moved with her husband to North Bay, until he died in 1948. She then returned to Bracebridge. Little is known about her activities at that time.

We do know that in 1952 she received several urgent letters from Godfrey A.P.V. Winter Baumgarten, postmarked Rome, imploring her to please try her

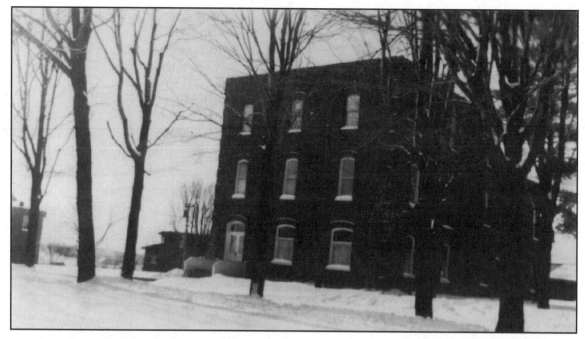

The Rene Caisse's Cancer Clinic, Bracebridge, Ontario, 1934 -1942. Sadly, this picture was taken after her famous clinic was shut down and hardly offers the scene of a "bustling, thriving, healing oasis" as described by numerous patients.

treatment on Eva Peron, wife of the Argentinian dictator, Juan Peron. She declined for reasons known only to herself.

For the most part until 1959 Rene remained out of sight. It was widely believed that she was still treating patients. Not surprising, given Rene's dedication to saving lives. One thing is for certain, the Commission had not forgotten about Rene. A letter written by C. J. Telfer, Secretary of the Commission for the Investigation of Cancer Remedies, to Dr. Mackinnon Phillips, Minister of Health, dated May 29, 1958, shows a continuing interest in her activities.

> "The nurse from Bracebridge who refused many years ago to divulge the formula is apparently still using it in the treatment of cancer. The Commission feels no action should be taken by them, but directed the matter be brought to your attention in case you might wish to refer this one also to the College of Physicians and Surgeons."

Dr. Phillips knew his history and did nothing, choosing, as it were, not to open Pandora's box.

But, even though Rene was not as active as she had been in the past, letters continued to arrive at the desk of Premier Leslie Frost from patients and supporters of Rene. Their content was always the same, former patients telling their stories of miraculous recoveries; supporters urgently requesting that Rene be allowed to "continue saving the lives of suffering humanity."

In September 1958 the Premier wrote to Rene. Here is an excerpt:

"It would speed matters up greatly if you would get in touch with Dr. W. G. Brown, Deputy Minister of Health, and arrange through him to give the Cancer Remedies Investigation Commission the details of your methods so the Commission could give them a thorough analysis."

The letter reflects a person who had absolutely no understanding of Rene or her past. One wonders if the Premier was joking or had been in a coma for the past 30 years. Did he seriously think Rene had somehow had a mysterious change of heart and would now simply turn over her Essiac formula to the Cancer Commission?

In January, 1959, it was apparent that Nurse Rene Caisse, 70, was still considered a threat to the Medical Establishment. Dr. M. B. Dymond, the Minister of Health, who (oddly) in the future would be involved with Essiac in a much different capacity, wrote to a supporter of Rene, R. J. Boyer, MPP for the Bracebridge area. Here in part is what he had to say:

"Dr. McPhedran assures me that the College will not prosecute (Rene) without first getting in touch with my deputy minister, or with me. I gathered, however, that it is their hope that Miss Caisse's activities might be controlled by means of surveillance, and that no prosecution would ever be necessary."

Essiac was not a dead issue – they were spying on her.

Rene's Triumphant Return

1959 marks a watershed in Rene's life. Although 70, she is about to begin what could arguably be the most important phase in the development of Essiac.

In February, 1959, a Canadian named Roland Davidson who had been cured by Essiac of a severe case of ulcerated hemorrhoids travelled to New York. His mission: to convince Ralph Daigh, Editorial Director and Vice President of Fawcett Publications (publisher of *True*, the world's largest men's magazine) that they should print the story of Rene Caisse and Essiac.

Roland Davidson had with him 30 years of documents, testimonials, letters from doctors, and newspaper articles, in all about 10 pounds of material which supported his story that a humble nurse from the back woods of Canada had stumbled onto a "cure for cancer."

Daigh, at first understandably highly skeptical, spent several hours going over Davidson's material. Gradually his skepticism gave way to sincere interest. Davidson had something! He took the material to his editor Douglas Kennedy, who after reviewing the material was equally impressed. But they knew if they published a story about a "natural" cure for cancer discovered by a "nurse" from Canada they had better be prepared to defend their story with real scientific data, not the hodge podge of materials Davidson had with him.

Daigh and a friend, Paul Murphy, of the Science Research Institute of New York, went to Bracebridge to interview Rene and several doctors who had worked with her. But Daigh had more in mind than just verifying Rene's story first hand. He brought along an agreement he would propose to Rene if he found Essiac worthy of further investigation. It was an agreement to go to Cambridge and work with one of the most prestigious doctors in the United States, Dr. Charles Brusch, MD.

Before going to Bracebridge Daigh had spoken to his friend Dr. Charles Brusch, who, after hearing the story, expressed keen interest in doing research on Essiac. Daigh believed if Essiac was thoroughly tested at the Brusch Clinic and subsequently earned Brusch's stamp of approval, it would be beyond reproach.

It didn't take much time in Bracebridge for both men to ascertain that Rene was sincere and Essiac did in fact have serious merit. They spoke to several doctors who had worked with Rene in the past. They reviewed patient records and chatted with some of Rene's old patients. All were very much alive and well. Rene and Essiac were real. They asked her if she would consider going to the Brusch Medical Center to do research on Essiac under the supervision of Dr. Charles Brusch.

Her expenses would be paid. She would retain the rights to her formula. She would be allowed to test Essiac on human cancer patients, and if testing proved positive, a corporation would be formed and Essiac would be made available to the public. It was exactly what Rene had wanted her entire adult life.

What did it matter that she was 70? What did it matter that she had been hounded for more than 30 years by an intransigent Medical Establishment? She believed it her destiny to bring "God's gift" into the hands of suffering humanity, and Dr. Brusch could be just the person to make it all possible.

She agreed to go to Cambridge. *(Fawcett Pub. never printed their story?)*

The Ultimate Partnership

Dr. Charles Brusch is one of the most respected physicians in the United States. He was President John F. Kennedy's personal doctor and trusted friend. His Curriculum Vitae, far too lengthy to include here, (See Appendix/ Exhibit 2, Page 103.) reads like the history of a national hero. His friends and colleagues include members of congress, the supreme court, the elite from every sector of society. Yet he possesses no airs, exhibits no elitism. Few human beings have collected the number of honors, awards and citations, bestowed on Dr. Brusch both as a physician and humanitarian. The Brusch Medical Center is one of the largest medical clinics in Massachusetts.

Why then would a physician of such note, held in *high* esteem by the Medical Establishment, the physician who administered the first polio vaccine in the United States, have an interest in working with a humble nurse from Canada who allegedly had an "unproven" cancer cure, and who had trouble with the authorities to boot? Why, indeed?

Although Dr. Brusch was highly respected by the Medical Establishment, he had his own ideas about the most effective ways to practice medicine. He

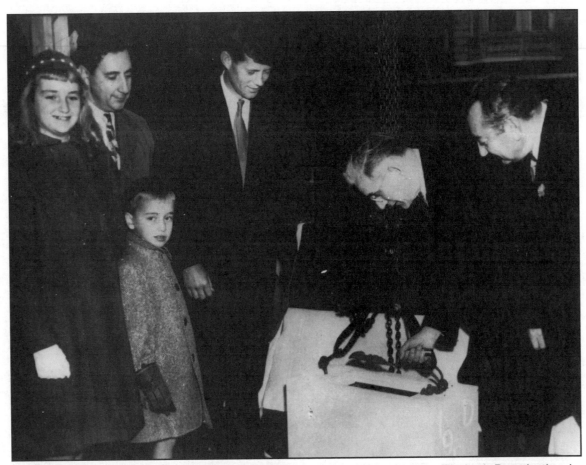

Laying the Corner Stone for the Brusch Medical Clinic. From the left. Mary Elizabeth Brusch, daughter, Dr. Charles Brusch M.D., John Brusch, son, President John F. Kennedy, at that time a Senator, John McCormack, Speaker of the House, and Dr. Joseph Brusch, brother.

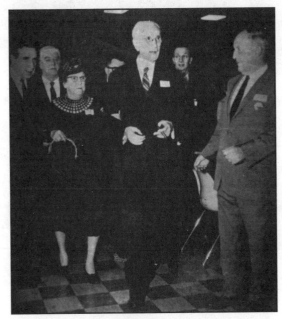

Dr. Charles Brusch (far left) is shown again with the well known former and late Speaker of the House, John W. McCormack of Massachusetts and Mrs. McCormack.

was by anyone's standards a unique human being. Dr. Brusch had studied acupuncture, had set up the first clinic to conduct acupuncture research, and was presently using it in his clinic when Rene arrived in 1959. Only a handful of doctors in the U.S. had heard of acupuncture, let alone used it as a regular form of treatment in 1959.

Dr. Brusch was the first doctor in the western hemisphere to initiate a plan in his clinic (similar to medicare) for people who did not have the money to pay for medical help. Nothing so earth shattering, but it was in 1959! Dr. Brusch's concern for suffering humanity was no less than Rene's.

It's also instructive to note that before Dr. Brusch was to become

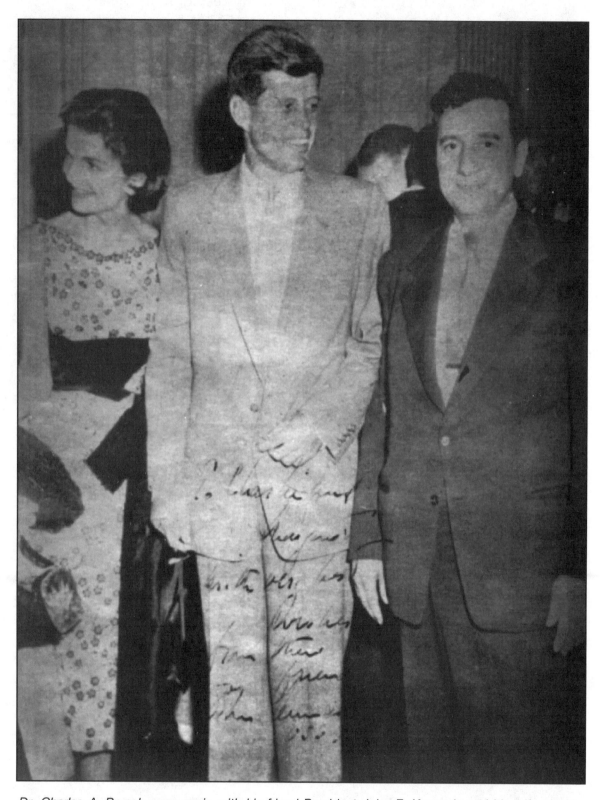

Dr. Charles A. Brusch once again with his friend President John F. Kennedy and his wife, Jackie. Inscription on the photograph reads: To Charlie and Margaret with very best wishes from your friend John Kennedy.

involved with Rene, he was already highly interested in preventive medicine, nutrition, and other forms of natural treatment. At a time when traditional medicine scoffed at even the idea that diet played some role in disease, that preventative therapy was an important part of medical practice, and that natural substances could be effective against certain diseases, Dr Brusch's thinking was heretical to say the least.

However, one of Dr. Brusch's greatest talents (and there were many) was his incredible ability to search for the truth with an open unbiased mind, while at the same time maintaining a respectful relationship, indeed receiving great accolades from the very people who had a reputation for stifling unorthodox thinking. The defenders of the status quo had met their match with Dr. Brusch. Believing he was one of them, they chose to support rather than destroy him.

Whether by providence or chance, Rene couldn't have found a better partner!

Rene arrived at the Brusch Clinic in May, 1959. She immediately went to work under the supervision of both Dr. Brusch and Dr. Charles McClure, Director of Research.

Her first patient was a 40 year old woman named Lena Burcell. X-rays showed her to be terminally ill with lung cancer. After receiving her first treatment with Essiac from Rene, she reported an immediate improvement in her ability to breathe. The severe pains she was experiencing in her joints lessened. She lived for three months.

A biopsy on a patient named John Cronin confirmed that he was terminally ill with cancer of the right lung. He took seven weekly treatments of Essiac at the Brusch clinic and the pains in his chest all but disappeared, along with his shortness of breath. He could now climb several flights of stairs without effort, and again took up his hobby of swimming.

Russell McCassey, suffering from basal cell carcinoma of the right cheek, proved by biopsy, was administered four Essiac treatments. The lesion changed colour from red to pale pink, and then reduced in size, markedly. The main ulcer crater formed by the cancer was observed to be disappearing.

Five weeks later the lesion was completely healed. Only a small scar remained, caused by the biopsy.

Wilbur Dymond, 58, suffered from prostate cancer. After just two months of treatment, all hardness had vanished, except for a single small nodule. He reported he no longer suffered excruciating pain during urination.

After just three months of treating patients with Essiac, Dr. Brusch and Dr. McClure were deeply impressed. In their first report about Essiac they wrote:

> "Clinically, on patients suffering from pathologically proven cancer, it reduces pain and causes a recession in the growth; patients have gained weight and shown an improvement in their general health.
>
> This after only three months' tests and the proof Miss Caisse has to show of the many patients she has benefited in the past 25 years, has con-

vinced the doctors at the Brusch Medical Center that Essiac has merit in the treatment of cancer. The doctors do not say that Essiac is a cure, but they do say it is of benefit. It is non-toxic, and is administered both orally and by intramuscular injection."

(See Appendix/ Exhibit 3, Page 105.)

Dr. Brusch encouraged Rene to also test Essiac on mice as well as clinically, not so much to see if it was effective (he had already seen convincing evidence it was) but also, as partners in research and development, to refine and perfect her formula by adding new herbs if required to obtain optimum results. This time Rene enthusiastically agreed. The Memorial Sloan-Kettering Institute in New York agreed to provide the mice. With the expert advice and scientific knowledge of Dr. Brusch they set about to discover as

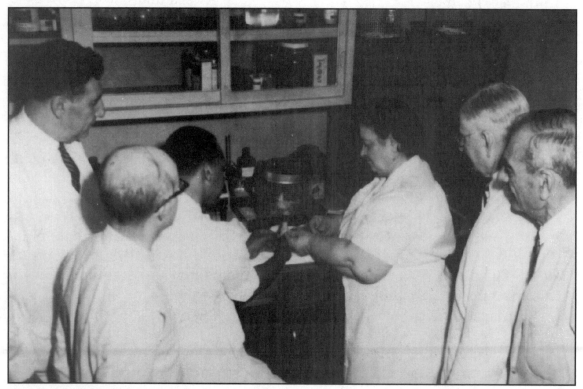

In the Laboratory at the Brusch Medical Center, Cambridge Massachusetts. Dr Brusch (far left) along with associates, looking on as Rene Caisse performs Lab. tests.

much as they could about the old Indian remedy. They were not disappointed.

According to Dr. Brusch, Dr. Philip Merker of the Memorial Sloan-Kettering Cancer Center did the autopsy surveys on the mice treated with Essiac. Dr. Merker observed definite and pronounced changes in the animals, which had not been found in the controls. They were very interested in further testing, but like his predecessors, would have to have the formula to establish if Essiac had any "real" merit in the treatment of cancer. Ever suspicious of the medical establishment, Rene refused.

The National Cancer Institute was also interested in testing Essiac, but like Sloan-Kettering, they wanted the formula. They were met with the same response from Rene. No!

It would appear that Dr. Brusch understood Rene's refusal because he never pushed the issue. The study of Essiac on both humans and mice would have to continue at the Brusch Clinic without the involvement of the venerated cancer institutions.

And continue it did. Dr. Brusch was no newcomer to the field of herbal medicine. Over the years he had developed a close relationship with Elmer Grove of Lathrop, Missouri, a master herbalist widely regarded as a great authority on the subject. With his help Dr. Brusch was able to perfect the original Essiac formula to such a degree it no longer needed to be injected. Dr. Brusch felt that injecting Essiac muscularly was an awkward and uncomfortable way to administer it. Furthermore it wasn't feasible for some cancer sufferers.

What they discovered through extensive experimentation on human patients was that by adding more herbs (called *potentiators**) to Essiac's original *core* formula, Essiac became even more effective. So much so that it was possible to administer the entire formulation orally. This was quite a breakthrough because it meant that people could treat themselves in the privacy of their own homes. Long treks to the clinic were no longer necessary. Especially good news to those patients who either couldn't afford transportation or were in such pain they couldn't bear to travel. Essiac in its newly evolved formulation was never again administered by injection to human patients.

During the course of their research, Dr. McClure decided to send out questionnaires to some of Rene's former patients to determine their long term survival rate. He received back a number of testimonials, all properly witnessed, that seemed to reflect what Rene had always maintained: Essiac cured cancer:

Norma Thompson	treated 20 years ago.	No recurrence. Alive and well.
Clara Thornbury	treated 22 years ago.	No recurrence. Alive and well.
DH Laundry	treated 11 years ago.	No recurrence. Alive and well.
Nellie McVittie	treated 23 years ago.	No recurrence. Alive and well.
Wilson Hammer	treated 31 years ago.	No recurrence. Alive and well.
John McNee	treated 30 years ago.	No recurrence. Alive and well.
Jack Finley	treated 20 years ago.	No recurrence. Alive and well.
Lizzie Ward	treated 14 years ago.	No recurrence. Alive and well.
JH Stewart	treated 16 years ago.	No recurrence. Alive and well.
Eliza Veitch	treated 18 years ago.	No recurrence. Alive and well.
Fred Walker	treated 20 years ago.	No recurrence. Alive and well.

Rene's life couldn't have been going better. She and Dr. Brusch through careful study, observation, and experimentation had perfected the original Essiac formula to a degree that left little question as to its effectiveness – *she thought*. But once again the Medical Establishment found its way into Rene's life. The labs supplying the inoculated mice suddenly stopped supplying them. In a letter written to Dr. Brusch they said:

*(*Potentiate: to cause to be more potent, to increases the effectiveness of.)*

"We cannot send you a report along the outline requested, for obvious reasons. *(What were the obvious reasons?)* We also regret to inform you that because of technical difficulties, we will be unable to process similar material in the future."

Something had happened. Compounding the problem, the American Medical Association (mother of all Establishments) made it clear to Dr. Brusch and Rene that it forbade its members to refer patients to unknown remedies. Thus the number of available patients dramatically dropped.

Rather than get into another battle Rene chose to go home. She felt she had accomplished what she had set out to do. She had been given the opportunity to test Essiac under the conditions she had always desired. She had been able to work with one of the most prestigious doctors in the United States. She felt Essiac's effectiveness against cancer and other health problems had been so clearly proven and demonstrated that no one could now doubt its merit. *Wishful thinking perhaps.*

Furthermore she had formed a deep friendship and a legal partnership with Dr. Brusch. A partnership that guaranteed Rene that Dr. Brusch would continue to research and perfect Essiac, and, if they eventually thought it viable, market it to the general public at a reasonable price.

She respected and trusted Dr. Brusch completely and was sure her formula was safe in his hands. History will prove she was correct.

Rene reluctantly returned to Bracebridge. Dr. Brusch, as promised, continued to work with Essiac when he could, both on patients and in the laboratory.

In 1984 Dr. Brusch was to give Essiac his ultimate vote of confidence by treating his own cancer solely with Essiac.

In his words written in 1990:

"I endorse this therapy even today for I have in fact cured my own cancer, the original site of which was the lower bowel, through Essiac alone. In my last complete examination, where I was examined throughout the intestinal tract while hospitalized (August, 1989) for a hernia problem, no sign of malignancy was found. Medical documents validate this.

I have taken Essiac every day since my diagnosis (1984) and my recent examination has given me a clean bill of health. I remained a partner of Rene Caisse until her death in 1978 and was the only person who had her complete trust and to whom she confided her knowledge and 'know-how' of what she named Essiac."

(See Appendix/ Exhibit 4, Page 107.)

The Latter Years

From 1962 to 1978 Rene remained active in Bracebridge. She continued to supply Essiac to Dr. Brusch who in turn continued to experiment, and perfect the original formula. He always kept her updated as to his progress and what additions he had made to the original formula. He also informed her periodically as to the other conditions he observed Essiac benefiting, such as diabetes and conditions due to high levels of toxicity. Essiac proved to be a phenomenal detoxifier.

In Canada, Essiac remained alive by word of mouth. People from all over the country somehow found their way to Rene. But she was getting old and she was tired. Still fearing the ever-watchful eyes of the Cancer Commission, she tried to secretly help as many as she could, but inevitably she would have to turn some away. It broke her heart.

No one has ever fully understood why, in 1973, when you take into consideration Rene's past experiences with the Medical Establishment, she decided to give them one more try. She was 85 years old in 1973, but apparently had not given up all hope that her old nemesis might be ready to reconsider.

She wrote to Sloan-Kettering and asked them if they would like to continue the encouraging tests they had done in 1959. Dr. Chester Stock, vice president and associate director of administrative and academic affairs, said they would definitely begin running tests on mice if Rene would send some Essiac.

Rene did in fact over the next three years send material to be injected into mice. But the mice it seems were implanted with animal carcinoma. Rene believed the mice would be implanted with human carcinoma. When she found out, she suspected Sloan-Kettering's test methods and the lab reports. When she received more disappointing lab results she was further convinced that the serum was being prepared improperly, "not in accordance with her directions." She even felt that some of the lab reports she received were actually not from the Sloan-Kettering's labs. *(?)* In 1976 she stopped sending them material, and terminated her agreement with Dr. Stock.

According to Dr. Stock, for mice to be implanted with human cancer, they must be so thoroughly irradiated that tests are sometimes inconclusive. But even though the new tests with Essiac proved inconclusive, he believed that there are always species differences, and didn't rule out the possibility that Essiac might be effective against human cancer.

But here's where it gets confusing. The material Rene sent to Dr. Stock was 25 years old, and she only sent one herb, the injectable one. She never mentioned the fact that Essiac had been further perfected at the Brusch Clinic. Nor did she ever send him the complete formula, or the other herbs so vital to Essiac's effectiveness. *(?)*

In an interview with *Homemaker's* Magazine in 1977 Dr. Stock stated:

> "He would be willing to do further testing if Rene would send the complete formula with its ingredients, so he could follow the injection with the oral brew."

Her own words at that time leave no doubt as to how she felt about the tests at Sloan-Kettering:

"Last time, they froze it. They might as well have been injecting distilled water!"

But why didn't Rene at least send the complete herbs necessary to get accurate results? She would not have had to reveal the exact formula. After all, it was Rene who initiated the new relationship with Sloan-Kettering.

Are we forced to conclude that Rene subconsciously had no real intention of cooperating with the Medical Establishment, given her past experiences? Or did she feel, possibly on a conscious level, the need to make a final perfunctory effort with the powers that be? We'll never know.

Her Final Act

In the summer of 1977 Rene was back in the limelight. She was 89.

After much initial skepticism and careful investigation, *Homemakers* Magazine in Canada released an extensive story on the entire history of Rene and Essiac. They opened their story with the following statement:

> "Essentially, Rene's story was true. She had been getting remarkable results against many kinds of cancer with Essiac, and she had been prevented from carrying on treatment unless she revealed the formula. Whether it would have been swept under the rug by a jealous medical hierarchy, as she feared, or hailed by a grateful profession that heaped honors at her door, is a question that no one can answer, since Essiac never stood the test of controlled clinical studies."

The management of *Homemakers* were so impressed with what they discovered during the course of their very thorough investigation that they made an official proposal to Rene, which they wrote about:

> "In the hope that we might speed Essiac on its way through the bureaucratic maze with no more loss of time, we offered to set up a trust to represent her in any dealings she might have with the government, Cancer Institute or any interested pharmaceutical companies."

Rene, never telling *Homemakers* about her existing partnership with Dr. Brusch, flatly turned them down. A disappointed *Homemaker's* concluded:

> "There's a tragic and shameful irony in the Essiac tale. In the beginning, a simple herbal recipe was freely shared by an Indian who understood that the blessings of the Creator belong to all.
>
> In the hands of more sophisticated (and allegedly more 'civilized') healers, it was made the focus of an ugly struggle for ownership and power. Perhaps our cure for cancer lies back in the past, with our discarded humility and innocence. Perhaps the Indians will someday revive an old man's wisdom, and share it once again. Perhaps this story will be the catalyst; if so, our efforts will not have been in vain."

Homemaker's Magazine is a widely read national publication. The story on Essiac in the summer of 1977 hit Canada like a nuclear bomb. It wasn't the first time, of course, that Canadians had heard about Rene and Essiac, but this story was different. It chronicled virtually every aspect of Essiac's tumultuous history. It was replete with testimonials and facts to back up every assertion about Essiac's incredible effectiveness. It gave the most clear picture to date of Rene and her lifelong struggle to have Essiac recognized as a legitimate cancer treatment.

Rene was swamped with requests for her treatment. Her phone rang non stop. Later a television crew came to Bracebridge and produced an hour long documentary on Rene. Newspapers across Canada picked up the story. Letters poured in. So intense was the attention that she was forced to accept police protection against the crowds of people swarming her house demanding she treat them with Essiac

Among the people influenced by *Homemaker's* story was David Fingard, a distinguished-looking 70 year old gentleman, vice president of Resperin, a Canadian corporation said to have pharmaceutical interests. Fingard couldn't believe that in over 50 years, no one had been able to capitalize on Essiac. No one had been able to wrestle the formula away from Rene? No one had been able to convince her that they could really do something big with this obvious medical breakthrough? He would be the one! He set out single handedly to obtain the formula.

When Fingard first approached Rene she as usual turned him down. But he was incredibly persistent. Nearly every day he arrived at her house with a new proposal. He told her Resperin, if granted the formula, would only test Essiac on humans. Another day he told her Resperin was backed by Dennison Mines, a large Canadian mining company, and therefore would have the capital to do anything necessary to bring Essiac to "suffering humanity." Yet another day he told her she could be directly involved in the future development of Essiac. Rene refused every offer. Fingard didn't give up. As a businessman he knew Essiac's potential.

Finally Fingard proposed something even Rene could not turn down. He told Rene if she granted Resperin the exclusive rights to the formula, Resperin would open five fully staffed clinics across Canada and give Essiac free to terminally ill cancer patients who couldn't afford its modest proposed price. She was interested.

Rene discussed the offer with her partner, Dr. Brusch. He agreed with her that Resperin's offer went beyond what any other person or company had proposed to date. There had been many offers in the past but she felt virtually all of them simply wanted to exploit Essiac. Something neither Rene nor Dr. Brusch would ever allow. Fingard's offer sounded different. Dr. Brusch went to meet Rene to formally co-sign the contract as partners.

On the morning of Oct. 26, 1977, David Fingard, Dr. Brusch and Rene met. Everybody was in a positive mood, it was a lovely autumn day, cool and crisp. The dappled orange and red trees that lined the quiet Bracebridge streets announced the coming of a new season.

Fingard handed Rene and Dr. Brusch the contract. It stated that Rene and her partner Dr. Brusch would receive $1 for signing and $250 per week for six months while Essiac was being tested. Out of the $250 Rene was to buy the herbs and prepare the formula for Resperin, who would then test it in a scientifically controlled study on humans. If the test proved positive, Essiac would subsequently be marketed to the general public. Rene and Dr. Brusch would receive a two percent royalty. (See Appendix/ Exhibit 5, Page 109.)

Dr. Brusch was shocked! There was so little money for Rene, who lived so modestly! He told Rene that she should take the entire amount, and if something came of Resperin's test they would then split the royalty. Rene, not at all concerned about the paltry sum offered by Fingard, or the fact that she would have to buy the herbs out of her tiny payments *(and prepare the herbs for Resperin!)* left to get the formula. Her purpose as it had always been was to get Essiac into the hands of suffering humanity. Fingard had convinced her that Resperin could make it happen. She was not going to let the question of her compensation spoil what was surely her last opportunity to save countless lives.

When Rene returned she signed the contract (Dr. Brusch signed it only as a witness that day) and then handed Fingard, who was waiting patiently, a sealed enveloped which she said contained "the formula." Everyone shook hands. Fingard left thoroughly pleased with his accomplishment.

He had done the impossible. He had done what no one had done before him. He had the exclusive rights to Essiac, a product that would certainly make him and his company rich beyond his wildest dreams.

Shortly after, Resperin applied to the Department of Health and Welfare asking permission for "Essiac" to be tested in a pilot program on terminal cancer patients. Officially the program was classified as a preclinical new drug submission, regulated by the Health Protection Branch of the Department of Health and Welfare. Hundreds of doctors across Canada, plus two hospitals, were to administer Essiac to their patients and monitor the results which would then be compiled by Resperin with the intention of getting Essiac eventually approved for widespread use as a legitimate cancer treatment.

Because of *Homemaker's* recent story, there was a tremendous amount of public pressure on the Department of Health and Welfare to get Essiac out to the public. After some delay, they granted Resperin's request to begin testing, as long as they adhered to the guidelines set forth by the Department of Health and Welfare.

The formula Rene gave Resperin was officially registered with the Department of Health and Welfare as ESSIAC, an experimental drug available for treatment of terminal cancer patients with approval from the Health Protection Branch of the Department of Health and Welfare.

The public was thrilled. Resperin was wildly positive about the future. Dr. P. B. Rynard, the Resperin chairman (in name only!) and a Canadian MP, was quoted as saying:

> "They looked carefully at all the facts, reviewed case histories which were very helpful. And one thing they discovered is that it

wasn't toxic in any way... there is no doubt that Essiac is effective for some types of cancer."

David Fingard was more effusive:

> "Essiac is one of the greatest discoveries in modern science. We have found certified cases of cancer ranging over a period of 25 to 30 years which have been cured by Essiac."

Several months later, it was apparent that something was amiss. Things were going much slower than planned. The two hospitals that had agreed to work with Resperin wanted to change the agreed-upon protocol for testing Essiac. Instead of using Essiac as a single and sole treatment to test on terminal cancer patients, they now wanted to use Essiac in combination with other therapies deemed appropriate by the attending physicians. In other words if a doctor determined that chemotherapy or radiation was appropriate for a patient, it would then be administered along with Essiac. This of course would skew the results, making it impossible to determine the effectiveness of Essiac.

The Medical Establishment was up to its same old games. If the treatment *worked* they could claim it worked because of the other therapies employed and not Essiac, as they had done during the Cancer Commission hearings. If the treatment did *not* work they could simply blame it on Essiac, and not on the damage done by conventional therapies, as they had also done during those same hearings.

Resperin may have been able to secure permission to test Essiac but it was a long way from getting any real cooperation from the Medical Establishment. The Health Protection Branch decided not to use the two hospitals. The clinical testing of Essiac would be limited to the private physicians participating in the test.

However, the situation with the private doctors was not much better. Many of the doctors, although enthusiastic about the possibilities of Essiac, were reluctant to comply with the stringent guidelines set forth by the Department of Health and Welfare for clinical testing of Essiac. The stage was set for a major debacle. (See Appendix/ Exhibit 6, Page 111.)

Rene complained publicly whenever she could:

> "I think I was able to accomplish more myself!"

Why wasn't the testing going forth as planned? Why weren't her five clinics being opened like Resperin had promised? Not fully understanding the circumstances, Rene blamed Resperin for the delay. She was bitterly disappointed.

She had fought valiantly for more than 50 years to bring Essiac to suffering humanity, resisting all temptation to capitalize on what was truly a gift from God. She had sacrificed everything – her personal life, her comfort, her peace of mind in her waning years. She had endured for most of her adult life the constant threat of imprisonment, censure and ridicule from a closed-minded, all too powerful Medical Establishment whose primary concern was not *healing,* but that their authority to dictate *how* people should be healed never be questioned under any circumstances.

For the time being the Medical Establishment had won the battle. Rene could fight no more. It would now be up to her successors to carry on the war.

On December 26th, 1978, Rene died from complications suffered after being operated on a week earlier to mend a broken hip. She was buried in a cemetery near Bracebridge. Her funeral on a cold winter day was attended by hundreds of mourners from not only Canada but around the world.

The extraordinary life of "Saint" Rene was over, but her dream to somehow bring Essiac to suffering humanity would in a few short years become a reality.

The fulfillment of Rene's dream will be the subject of *Section Two.*

Section Two

The Torch Is Passed
– Essiac's Evolution –
1978-1992

Synchronicity: Meaningful coincidence, significantly related patterns of chance.

A Golden Opportunity

In 1982 the Department of Health and Welfare shut down the clinical testing program for Essiac, accusing Resperin of conducting a flawed and worthless investigation.

As it turned out Resperin had actually provided the Medical Establishment with a golden opportunity, an opportunity they had been unable to secure since they first declared war on Essiac more than 50 years before.

But to understand exactly what that opportunity was, it is important to first understand the Resperin Corporation in more detail.

Who was Resperin? A question that in early 1980 was very much on the mind of Dr. Brusch. It seems his grave misgivings about David Fingard and Resperin were to prove correct.

After entering into the agreement with Resperin, Dr. Brusch was kept totally in the dark as to the progress of the Essiac testing program, or anything else concerning Essiac. His phone calls were not returned, his correspondence remained unanswered. This in spite of the fact that his contract with Resperin clearly stated that he would be regularly consulted and kept abreast of all details about the testing and subsequent marketing of Essiac.

Rene was gone so Dr. Brusch really had no way to find out what was happening in Canada unless he heard from Resperin. He was frustrated, angry and worried. Finally, Dr. Brusch hired a private investigator to try and determine the status of the testing, and just who in fact Resperin really was. It was an action (he was later to comment} that he should have taken before even considering involvement with Resperin.

The investigation led to some rather startling discoveries. First and foremost was the fact that Resperin was at the time of *Homemaker's* article not a viable corporation. It was out of business for all practical purposes, and had been for some time. During its tenure, the length of which was unclear, Resperin had sold some type of respiratory products, but what those products were and who they were sold to was also unclear. Resperin did have an impressive board of advisors, but they were all unpaid consultants and friends of David Fingard, charmer that he was.

As for David Fingard the investigation verified that he was a trained chemist, but where his expertise lay was anybody's guess. The Resperin Laboratory where Essiac was said to be formulated after Rene's death turned out to be the kitchen of Dr. Matthew Dymond who was the only other Resperin employee. He and his wife filled prescriptions literally by brewing batches of the Essiac tea the night before on their kitchen stove.

Dr. Matthew Dymond had been in fact the Minister of Health. He was a prominent medical doctor and there is no reason to doubt his credentials or his medical knowledge. The fact that he had been a Minister of Health had surely helped Resperin secure it's clinical testing permit. But both men were now in their seventies. Their dream to resurrect Resperin for the express purpose of someday cashing in on Essiac's very real potential, was just that. A dream. Both aging gentlemen had neither the strength, discipline, time nor money to actualize their fantasy.

Obviously, Resperin was hardly the pharmaceutical powerhouse Fingard had represented it to be. Nowhere was there any indication of large financial backing from Dennison Mines, or anybody else. The only real power Resperin had was the unquestionably persuasive power of David Fingard. And Fingard had applied that power with notable skill, fooling both Rene and Dr. Brusch, among others.

The testing that had been been conducted for a year and a half by Resperin with private physicians was not going as planned to say the least. Some doctors were actually unable to get supplies of Essiac from Resperin when they needed them. The batch composition was uncontrolled and would differ from week to week, few records were kept as to patient progress, and virtually none of the doctors conducting clinical trials were closely monitored by Resperin. Not surprising, considering Resperin's resources and the age of its principals!

Unfortunately, as previously stated, the debacle that was unfolding played right into the hands of the Medical Authorities. They finally had Essiac right where they wanted it. Resperin had unwittingly made it possible for the

Department of Health and Welfare to discredit Essiac in a manner they had never been able to in the past. The Department of Health and Welfare had a plan: it would be a three pronged attack. Their devious strategy was well conceived, and they executed it with precision.

On April 9, 1981, the Health Protection Branch wrote the following internal briefing memorandum to clarify to its members the intended future actions it would take against Resperin:

> Essiac, a herbal product intended for treatment of cancer and produced by the Resperin Corporation, was conditionally cleared for clinical trials in 1978. At that time, the Health Protection Branch took no objection to the distribution of Essiac to qualified investigators for the purpose of clinical testing to obtain evidence with respect *to its safety, dosage and effectiveness.* This decision was based on the understanding that Essiac would be manufactured under appropriate controls as required by the Food and Drug Regulations and that the clinical trials with Essiac would be monitored by a national agency concerned with cancer therapy, *in order to arrive at scientifically valid data to substantiate the effectiveness of this drug in treatment of malignant disease(s).*
>
> In spite of repeated reminders from the Health Protection Branch, the drug manufacturer failed to implement the above conditions. Essiac was distributed by the Resperin Corporation to some 160 physicians throughout Canada for treatment of cancer patients.
>
> To date, the Health Protection Branch has received a small number of incomplete clinical case reports, but no data which would establish that the product distributed is uniform in composition from batch to batch. Without this information, the results of the clinical studies *are impossible to evaluate.* Concerns about the clinical use of Essiac and the diversion of patients from proven conventional methods of therapy have been repeatedly expressed by members of the medical profession.
>
> The data presently available on Essiac were recently reviewed independently by two nongovernment consultants, known medical specialists on cancer treatment. *Both consultants found the clinical studies poorly conceived and executed, yielding uninterpretable results.* Termination of the clinical trials as currently constituted was recommended by both consultants.
>
> In view of this, the Health Protection Branch, on behalf of the Minister, pursuant to Section C. 08. 005 (3) intends to notify the Resperin Corporation that in the interest of public health, the clearance of the investigational new drug submission for Essiac will be cancelled.
>
> It can be expected that this decision will give rise to some accusations that the medical establishment is not prepared to give the drug manufacturer a proper opportunity to establish its therapeutic value. There may also be a negative reaction from cancer victims who are presently taking Essiac and will have their supply cut off. Conversely, the decision will still criticism from the medical profession that the Branch is allowing an unproven drug to be distributed under inappropriate conditions.

(See Appendix/ Exhibit 7, Page 113.)

The Health Protection Branch had established a credible and legal reason to shut down Resperin's clinical trails. It was true that Resperin was conducting a shoddy test. No questions on that score. On August 30, 1982, the Minister of Health and Welfare, Monique Bégin, wrote to Resperin Corporation and informed them that the Department of Health and Welfare was terminating their permit for clinical testing of Essiac. The letter (See Appendix/ Exhibit 8, Page 115.) cites the reasons previously outlined in the internal memorandum to justify their actions. Resperin put up very little resistance. The reality of their undertaking had become all too apparent to the quixotic duo.

Numerous patients involved in the Essiac clinical trials vehemently protested the decision to stop testing Essiac. For them it was a matter of life or death!

But the Department of Health and Welfare had predicted a firestorm. They were prepared.

They magnanimously informed the public that they would allow Essiac to be obtained under the Emergency Drug Release Act, virtually a public relations program for the Department of Health and Welfare that ostensibly provided unapproved medications for sufferers of terminal diseases, for "compassionate reasons." If a patient were diagnosed as having terminal cancer, he then could obtain Essiac with an *official* recommendation from his doctor. What was not revealed was that the maze of bureaucratic red tape which accompanied the Emergency Drug Release Act was more than most doctors were willing to go through to obtain Essiac for their patients. (See Appendix/ Exhibit 9, Page 117.)

The third and most important part of Department of Health and Welfare's plan to discredit Essiac was to lie to the public about their reasons for discontinuing the Resperin testing. If the public asked why the testing of Essiac had been cancelled they were given the following statement of so called facts:

> The Department of Health and Welfare had permitted Resperin to investigate Essiac in cancer patients at the Princess Margaret Hospital and the Toronto General Hospital. However the study was never done as neither of the two centers were willing to treat their cancer patients with Essiac alone. Instead, a decision was made by the Department to allow family practitioners to supervise Essiac treatment for terminal cancer patients.
>
> One hundred twelve physicians who had received Essiac under these circumstances were asked to submit case reports. Seventy four responded on 87 cancer patients. Of these, 78 showed no benefit. Investigation of the nine remaining cases revealed that the cancer was progressing (four cases), the patient had died (two cases) or the patients had previously undergone some form of cancer treatment which could have stabilized the disease. *From the data collected,* it was concluded that Essiac did not alter the progress of cancer and the pre-clinical New Drug Submission was subsequently revoked.
>
> No clinical evidence exists to support claims that Essiac is an effective treatment for cancer. For this reason, Health and Welfare Canada does not permit it to be marketed as a drug.

At the same time, it is acknowledged that Essiac is not harmful to a person's health providing it is not substituted for *proven* forms of cancer therapy. In fact, there may be positive psychological effects for some cancer patients. In recognition of this, Health and Welfare Canada has historically authorized emergency release of Essiac on compassionate grounds.

(Proof of their deep concern for public health!)

And there you have it. No question about it. Essiac had a real chance under clinical conditions to be tested on humans and failed miserably. More than a hundred physicians conducted clinical tests on Essiac. The data was collected and guess what – Essiac doesn't work! In fact the statistics are almost identical to what the Cancer Commission found on other patients back in 1939. It didn't work on almost all of the patients then, and if a patient happened to get better, it was only attributable to traditional therapies the patient had taken previously, or to wrong diagnoses. And the same thing is true today. Imagine that.

One slight problem exists however, which was never pointed out to the public. It would have been impossible to determine if Essiac was ineffective, as claimed by the Department of Health and Welfare, because by its own admission the Department of Health and Welfare had already categorically stated in their internal memorandum of 1981 that they found that "the results of the clinical studies are impossible to evaluate," moreover the clinical studies were "poorly conceived and executed, yielding uninterpretable results."

Resperin's permit to test Essiac was not revoked because Essiac was shown to be ineffective, but rather because the test to determine its effectiveness was flawed from the beginning! Resperin never once protested the flagrant abuse of truth perpetrated by the Medical Establishment, because to do so would have been tantamount to admitting to their own incompetence, something Fingard's enormous ego would never allow.

But the most damning contradiction to the Medical Establishments campaign to discredit Essiac came from one of its own members!

On October 5, 1983, E. Bruce Hendrick, M.D. (Chief of Neurosurgery at the Hospital for Sick Children at the University of Toronto – one of the most prestigious hospitals *and* physicians in all of Canada), wrote the following to Monique Bégin, Minister of Health and Welfare:

Dear Mme. Bégin:

I am writing this letter in support of a scientific clinical trial of the cancer treatment with the compound known as "Essiac."

At the present time, at the Hospital for Sick Children, there are some 10 patients with surgically treated tumors of the central nervous system, who have escaped from conventional methods of therapy including *both radiation and chemotherapy.*

The patients who were started on Essiac have, at the present time, too limited of a follow up period to reach a definite conclusion.

However, in eight of the ten patients, there has been significant improvement in their neurological state. For further confirmation of the effectiveness of this treatment we'll wait on CAT scans and subsequent investigation.

I am however most impressed with the *effectiveness of the treatment* and its lack of side effects.

I feel that this method of treatment should be given serious consideration and would benefit from a scientific clinical trial. Yours sincerely,

E. Bruce Hendrick, M.D., FRCS (c)
Chief, Division of Neurosurgery. (See Appendix/ Exhibit 10, Page 119.)

It seems the good doctor had been conducting his own test unbeknownst to the Department of Health and Welfare.

Not to worry. The letter was never revealed to the public.

For all practical purposes, at least in the collective brains of the Medical Establishment, Essiac was no longer a threat to their monopoly on cancer treatment. Their authority to dictate what healed and what didn't remained firmly intact. They were, however, unaware of another rebel in their camp – Dr. Brusch, who was still very much determined to see Rene's dream fulfilled. He would get his chance!

After Resperin's testing program was cancelled Resperin, for the most part, returned from whence it had come... retirement. The once boisterous Fingard was all but silenced. Resperin still made Essiac available for doctors who requested it under the Emergency Drug Release Program, but that took very little effort. Not much was requested, in large part due to the Department of Health and Welfare's successful campaign to discredit Essiac, coupled with the difficult requirements attached to obtaining it under the Emergency Drug Releases Program. Of the small amount of people whose doctors tried to obtain Essiac for them, 25 percent were turned down because they did not "qualify" for the program. Never mind that they were already pronounced terminal by a qualified physician.

Dr. Brusch finally gave up on Resperin realizing it consisted of little more than the pipe dreams of an aging Fingard and his equally aging associates.

There were several attempts by American companies to jump on board but this time Dr. Brusch did his homework. None of the offers had real merit. They were usually made by fast-buck artists or dreamers, or people with honorable intentions but no capital.

In the meantime, Dr. Brusch continued to use Essiac in his clinic with impressive results (as previously stated); even curing himself of cancer with it in 1984. He, of course, was convinced more than ever that he must somehow find a way to get Essiac into the hands of the public, but he was equally convinced that he would have to travel an entirely different path. His investigation of Resperin and their subsequent troubles with the Medical Establishment had made Dr. Brusch certain that any attempt to get Essiac approved as a drug would be next to impossible.

Maybe Rene and he had missed the obvious all those years. Maybe it had been unwise if not foolish to fight the Medical Establishment. Maybe there was a different way. That way would present itself in the person of Elaine Alexander.

Elaine Alexander

In 1984, Dr. Brusch received a phone call from a woman in Vancouver, British Columbia. She identified herself as "Elaine Alexander," a radio talk show host and producer. She explained to Dr. Brusch that she was interested in doing a radio series on Essiac, had already thoroughly researched the subject, and would like to do an "on the air interview" with him.

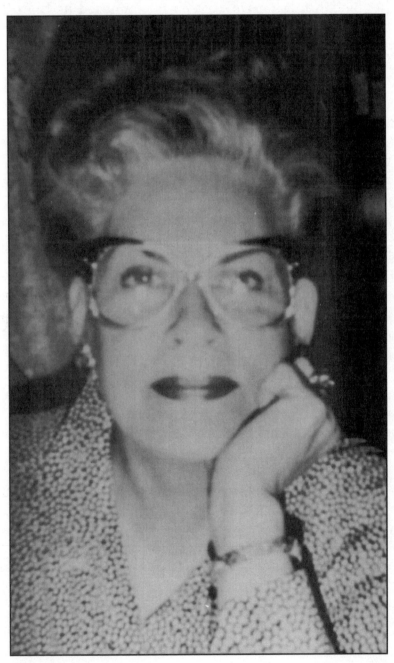

Elaine Alexander in 1993.

She told Dr. Brusch she had been a radio producer for 20 years, connected with shows "always known for their pioneering probing of many varied issues of importance – issues that are now taken for granted!" Recently she had started a new program called "Stayin' Alive." She was both the broadcaster and the producer.

Her new show was dedicated to health issues and all their varied aspects. It was cutting edge, controversial and highly informative. For example, in 1984 she broadcast an in-depth six week series on a new and devastating health problem, AIDS. This, when most people knew very little about it. She brought on the air Dr. Luc Montagne, the

French discoverer of the AIDS virus, among other notable authorities from around the world.

Many of her guests presented information about credible alternative therapies which had been banned or oppressed by the Medical Establishment. She possessed a wide range of understanding about the entire health industry, well versed in all areas of the "alternative movement." But her show did not focus exclusively on alternative therapies or controversial issues. She also presented the views of orthodox medical science and had as her guests many leading physicians. She was not afraid to present any side of an issue no matter what the consequences.

From the moment they began talking Dr. Brusch was amazed at Elaine's depth of understanding of Rene Caisse and the entire history of Essiac. She had meticulously researched the subject and it showed. She had interviewed numerous people who had recovered from terminal cancer using Essiac alone. Many of them knew Rene personally, and from them she acquired a remarkable understanding of Rene Caisse. She had painstakingly gone through court records, newspaper archives, and any other source which might shed light on the subject. She was passionate, eloquent, and deeply committed to revealing the truth. She seemed to display the same enthusiasm and confidence about Essiac as Rene herself. In fact, there was an uncanny similarity in attitude; oddly, even in their personalities.

She of course knew that Dr. Brusch was Rene's partner and as such knew more about Essiac than any other living person. But she had not contacted Dr. Brusch until she was well prepared, because she thought he might be reluctant to go on the air unless he was convinced that the interviewer knew what they were talking about. Her hunch paid off. Dr Brusch agreed to be interviewed. It was a first. Dr. Brusch had never granted a public interview before, fearing the broadcaster would try to sensationalize the story, further damaging the credibility of Essiac. Apparently Elaine had assuaged his fears.

The first interview was held with Dr. Brusch in November, 1984. The interview lasted for two hours. It was in-depth, probing and to the point. This was *talk* radio so the public was encouraged to call in. As soon as Dr. Brusch began talking every line at the station was jammed and stayed that way until long after the end of the interview.

It's not hard to imagine why! Here was one of the most prestigious doctors in the United States, personal physician to JFK, telling the public in his calm and authoritative voice that he had definite, indisputable proof that Essiac, a harmless herbal tea, cured cancer!

Elaine:

"Dr. Brusch have you studied Essiac's effect on cancer patients under controlled conditions at your clinic?"

Dr. Brusch:

"Yes, I have!"

Elaine:

"Were the results significant, or were the results, as some medical professionals have asserted in the past, simply anecdotal?"

Dr. Brusch:

"Highly significant!"

Elaine:

"Does Essiac have any side effects?"

Dr. Brusch:

"None."

Elaine:

"Dr. Brusch, lets get right to the point. Are you saying Essiac can *help* people with cancer, or are you saying that Essiac is a *cure* for cancer?"

Dr. Brusch:

"I'm saying it's a cure!"

Elaine:

"Would you repeat that once more Dr. Brusch?"

Dr. Brusch:

"Yes, I would be glad to. Essiac is a cure for cancer. I've seen it reverse and eliminate cancers at such a progressed state that nothing medical science currently has could have accomplished similar results. I wouldn't have believed it myself had I not seen it with my own eyes. I feel very strongly that Essiac is the single most beneficial treatment for cancer today."

It was an incredible event. Never had Elaine experienced such a tremendous response from her audience concerning any subject or guest she had presented, including other alternative treatments for cancer. Her shows were extremely popular, but this was different. There was something magical about the chemistry between Dr. Brusch and Elaine. Something that really brought the Essiac story to life.

Before the end of the show several people had actually driven to the station and were waiting outside in hopes of having their questions answered. Obviously they had been unable to get through by telephone because of the jammed lines.

Over the next two years Elaine produced seven two hour shows on Essiac. Dr. Brusch was interviewed four more times. Each show concentrated on a different part of the Essiac story. She brought on several other guests, including many former terminal cancer patients, all alive and well years after being treated with Essiac, doctors, co-workers, anyone of importance connected with the story. Every guest further verified Dr. Brusch's certainty that Essiac was indeed a cure for cancer.

Something was happening. The public began to treat Elaine as if she were Rene herself. Letters from all over the continent arrived daily asking all manner of questions about Essiac. But what most of the inquirers wanted was advice about how to obtain Essiac.

The stories they told about their cancerous conditions and the treatments they had received at the hands of orthodox medicine were heart wrenching: The agony of chemotherapy, organs removed, limbs cut off, horrible radiation burns. People's lives devastated, given up as hopeless. They saw Essiac as their first real hope, a possible reprieve from their nightmarish, dwindling existence. They pleaded with Elaine to please help them somehow obtain Essiac. She was engulfed in an ocean of pain and suffering.

As always, after each show people would be waiting outside hoping to have another chance at asking a question, or catching a glimpse of Elaine.

Naturally Elaine became more and more involved with her audience. She grew to be an expert at sorting out the red tape for both doctors and patients who had requested Essiac under the Emergency Drug Release Act. But it was a long process and very few cancer victims were able to secure the treatment, many of them dying before their doctors had filled out enough papers to qualify for the program.

The stress on Elaine was enormous. Some people stricken with cancer had found out where Elaine lived, literally camping on her porch until she would give them counsel, which she always tried to do. Elaine, like Rene herself, was unwilling to turn anyone down if she could be of some assistance. She was in constant touch with Dr. Brusch asking for his advice whenever she thought it necessary.

Elaine has said that 1984, 85, and 86 were the hardest and saddest years of her life. She had known intellectually for some time that Modern Medicine was woefully inept at treating cancer. But now every fiber of her being was acutely aware of the incredible amount of suffering that existed because of modern medicine's abject inability to heal cancer.

She had to do something! She had an idea. It was exquisitely simple.

For the past several years she and Dr. Brusch had conferred frequently. Thus it was only natural that they would become both friends and confidants. Dr. Brusch had expressed to Elaine on a number of occasions that it was still his dream to bring Essiac to the public but he (as previously mentioned) had to find a new way. However, work at his own clinic had prevented Dr. Brusch from pursuing different avenues.

Early in 1988 Elaine told Dr. Brusch her idea. He was so impressed he asked on the spot if she would become his partner! He knew she had great contacts in the health community. He knew that Elaine, like Rene Caisse, had the same boundless energy and conviction about the benefits of Essiac, and the same caring and concern for suffering humanity. He now knew that if anyone could finally bring Essiac into the hands of the public it would be Elaine.

Her idea went something like this:

Forget about trying to get the Medical Establishment to legitimize Essiac. It hadn't worked and it never would. The very nature of treating cancer with Essiac, a harmless herbal tea, flew right in the face of all orthodox thinking. Namely, that the diseased body takes radical intervention in the form of poison, radiation, or surgery to alleviate or eliminate the disease. The entire edifice of Modern Medicine is built on a mountain of so called scientific evidence to support their belief about the nature and treatment of disease. Furthermore, the Medical Establishment has a limitless amount of power and money to support and enforce their beliefs. To disagree is to be instantly labeled as a quack, and thereby to cease to exist.

Why fight a war that can't be won? Why not take Essiac out of the arena of the Medical Establishment all together? How? By simply selling Essiac through health food stores as nothing more than what it actually is, a harmless herbal *detoxifying* tea. Make no claims.

Of course you could not call the tea Essiac. Any attempt at marketing Essiac as an herbal tea would most likely be stopped by the authorities because the name Essiac was so closely associated with cancer treatment. The name alone carried a claim: Cure for cancer! *A Department of Health and Welfare internal memorandum released through the freedom of information act later confirmed this assumption.* (See Appendix/ Exhibit 11, Page 121.)

Why not drop the name Essiac and simply call it an herbal detoxifying tea. The tea would still contain the exact perfected Essiac formula. Hadn't the old Indian called his remedy *a holy drink that purified the body*? Hadn't Dr. Brusch spoken of Essiac's phenomenal detoxifying properties? Hadn't patients who had been treated with Essiac spoken of its effects in purge-like terminology: increased urination and evacuation, discharges of great masses of cottage-cheese-like materials, feelings of light and energy re-entering the body, and a sense of restored cleanliness and purity?

To speak of Essiac as a cure for cancer was the same as speaking of it as a drug in the eyes of the medical authorities. And to offer a drug to the public, it must first be approved as a "legitimate" drug. Something the Medical authorities were obviously never going to allow. But the old Indian remedy never was a drug. Drugs are designed to block or change some function of the body. Essiac is, in fact, a natural substance that was always meant to simply purify and detoxify the body, not block or change its function in some unnatural way. Drugs are, by their very nature, toxic. Essiac is, by its very nature, non-toxic. And therein lies its real power. Essiac is the ultimate body purifier. Thus, the body, once it is cleansed of toxic disease-producing impurities, has the power to heal itself.

Why not put Essiac back on the path of its Ojibwa originators, the path of balance and purity. Naturally it would take some time to catch on, because the manufacturer would be barred from making any cancer curing claims whatsoever. But it would be perfectly acceptable to say that this incredible herbal detoxifying tea, should be taken for any disease condition because its natural cleansing properties support the body's own internal healing ability. The results would speak for themselves. Once people started using it word would indeed spread.

No more battles with the Medical Establishment. No more years of waiting, testing, proving, all for nothing. Elaine was certain that if they changed Essiac's name, made no claims, and simply touted its benefits as a great herbal detoxifying tea, the Medical Authorities would be hard pressed to take it off the market. As far as she knew, herbal teas were not viewed as a threat to the Medical Establishment!

It was beautiful. The public would now have instant access to Essiac. It could be sold cheaply and would be readily available.

But for Elaine, becoming Dr. Brusch's partner and dedicating herself to making Rene and Dr. Brusch's dream come true would probably mean an end to her radio career. To be sure, to become a partner of a man of Dr. Brusch's stature was an incredible honor. His offer carried great weight. But her career had brought vital, lifesaving information to millions of people over the years. It was a tough decision, but in the end she felt she could do more for people by making Essiac widely available than she could by continuing in radio. After much soul searching, Elaine agreed to join with Dr. Brusch as partners, and on Nov. 10, 1988, legal documents were officially signed. Dr. Brusch then passed over to Elaine the refined and perfected Essiac formula, *plus* a number of *additional herbal formulas* proven over the years to have substantive healing powers for various aliments, such as prostate and urinary disorders, and others researched and perfected by Dr. Brusch and Rene during their partnership.

To reconfirm their continued association, more recently (March 26, 1993) a further legal contract between Elaine and Dr. Brusch was consummated.

(See Appendix/ Exhibit 12, Page 123.)

Now that Elaine and Dr. Brusch were partners and had a plan, the next step was to find a suitable manufacturer to make the herbal tea. It wasn't easy. In the past, even though Rene and Dr. Brusch had treated thousands of people with Essiac, it was nothing compared to the scale they now envisioned.

Rene usually picked or grew the herbs herself. Now they would have to rely on commercial herb producers and manufacturers. The quality of the herbs was essential. They had to be organic; no chemicals, no pesticides. The drying and formulating had to be done with scrupulous precision as Rene and Dr. Brusch had done in the past. The exact proportions among the herbs were vital. Testing in Dr. Brusch's clinic had verified this.

The distribution would have to be accomplished on a massive scale. The packaging would have to be excellent, conveying as much as it could about the tea's powers of detoxification, but making no other claims. In short, they would have to find a health products manufacturer that not only displayed a keen sense of quality and skill, but also a sincere understanding and commitment to the true spirit of Essiac. A sense of understanding and commitment equal to the one shared by Elaine, Dr. Brusch and Rene herself. It would take nearly 4 years and a lot of investigation to find a manufacturer that possessed all of the afore-mentioned qualities. In mid 1992 their search came to an end. Flora Manufacturing and Distributing Ltd. was chosen.

Flora

To understand why Elaine chose Flora to manufacture Essiac it is first important to understand the origins of the company. We have said that the old

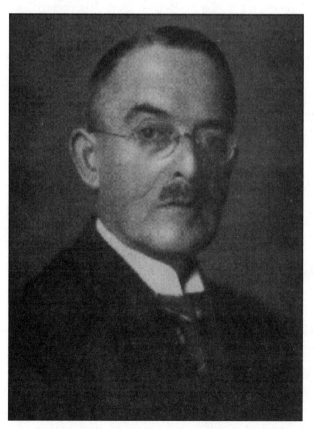

Indian remedy was described by the Ojibwa Indian medicine man as a "holy drink which purifies the body and places it back in balance with the great spirit." With that original description of Essiac in mind we will give you a brief synopsis of how Flora came into being and of its uncanny kinship to the ancient healing knowledge of the Ojibwa. There are no accidents.

In 1913 Dr. Otto Greither, grandfather of Thomas Greither (the director of Flora), lay gravely ill in a Bavarian hospital. At that time Dr. Greither was an orthodox medical doctor, believing completely in the dictates of his profession. Suddenly he had grown ill. His condition, which was impossible to diagnose, according to his colleagues, had left him paralyzed from the waist down. His legs had turned into hard, dark lifeless logs

Dr. Otto Greither M.D., the remarkable man who started the Greither health product Dynasty.

and one was starting to gangrene. He was advised by the best medical minds that his only hope to survive was amputation! On the eve of his operation a humble nurse *(another nurse!)* versed in traditional Bavarian folk ways of natural healing suggested to Dr. Greither that his condition was due to toxic build-up in his body, and that he need not undergo an operation to amputate his leg. His best remedy was to take a good *enema* to clean out his colon and alleviate the toxic build-up. Dr. Greither, at first scoffing at the nurse's suggestion, decided he had nothing to lose and took her advice. The effects were immediate. His operation was postponed and eventually cancelled after a series of daily enemas. In just a few weeks Dr. Greither was to return to his former life, healthy and robust with full use of his legs.

He was overjoyed at his recovery but still did not appreciate its full meaning. During the next six months he returned to his old life style, eating and drinking as he pleased. And again Dr. Greither was stricken and lost the use of his legs. And once again he underwent a regimen of enemas and regained his health. However, this time he fully grasped the importance of what had cured him. His healing experience had such a profound effect on him that he resolved to abandon his orthodox medical thinking and dedicate his life to natural healing. He changed his life style, becoming an ardent student of vegetarianism, and all forms of natural healing.

Dr. Greither discovered through his own experience and through his extensive research that most diseases (dis-ease) are a result of toxic build-up throughout the system, especially the colon. Once the body is in a toxic condition it is susceptible to any number of health problems, ranging all the way from cancer to a simple headache. If the body is stimulated naturally to cleanse itself, it will return in most cases to its natural state: radiant health. The body has miraculous healing powers but it has to be detoxified in order for it to make maximum use of its internal healing powers. Traditional medicine relied (and still relies) heavily on drugs. And although some drugs can alleviate symptoms, they very rarely if ever heal the body. Drugs can in fact, because of their toxicity, have the opposite effect and further damage an already compromised system.

In 1916 Dr. Otto Greither formed a company called Salus Haus (Health House) with the intention of producing high quality natural herbal tonics which would cleanse and purify the body. He was totally committed to producing the very best natural products in the world.

In just ten years he had more than 50 Salus Haus sales and information outlets throughout Germany, supplying an increasingly receptive public with his natural health products, particularly the Salus treatment, *an herbal detoxification drink.*

The company has continued to flourish ever since and has grown to one of the largest and most successful health product manufacturers in the world. Employing over 250 people, Salus Haus now owns organic fields throughout the fertile farming districts of Bavaria, an organic herbal farm in Chile, and an organic acerola farm in Florida. Its manufacturing facilities spanning more than 60 acres just outside Munich located in the picturesque German Black Forest have been voted the most advanced in all of Europe. Salus Haus products are exported to 60 countries and are known across the globe as simply the very best health products on the market today for naturally cleansing and revitalizing the body.

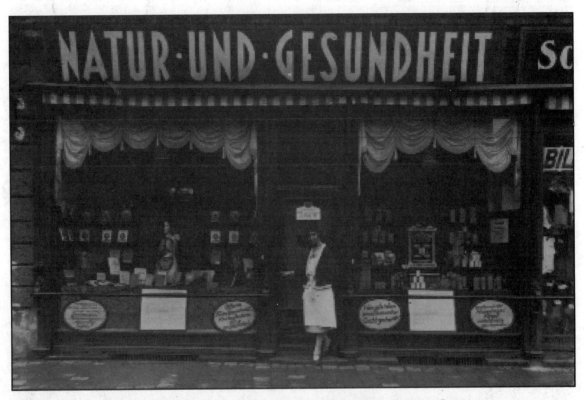

One of the first Salus Haus health food stores, approximately 1925, Bavaria, Germany.

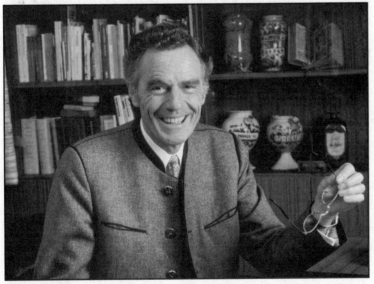

Otto Greither Jr,. Proprietor and Managing Director of Salus Haus today.

The Greither family has become what can only be described as a dynasty in the health products industry. Salus Haus is now headed by the son of Dr. Otto Greither, Otto Greither Jr. He in turn has three sons, all of whom have their own health product companies, located in Germany, Switzerland and Canada. All three of Otto Jr.'s sons own companies which are completely independent of

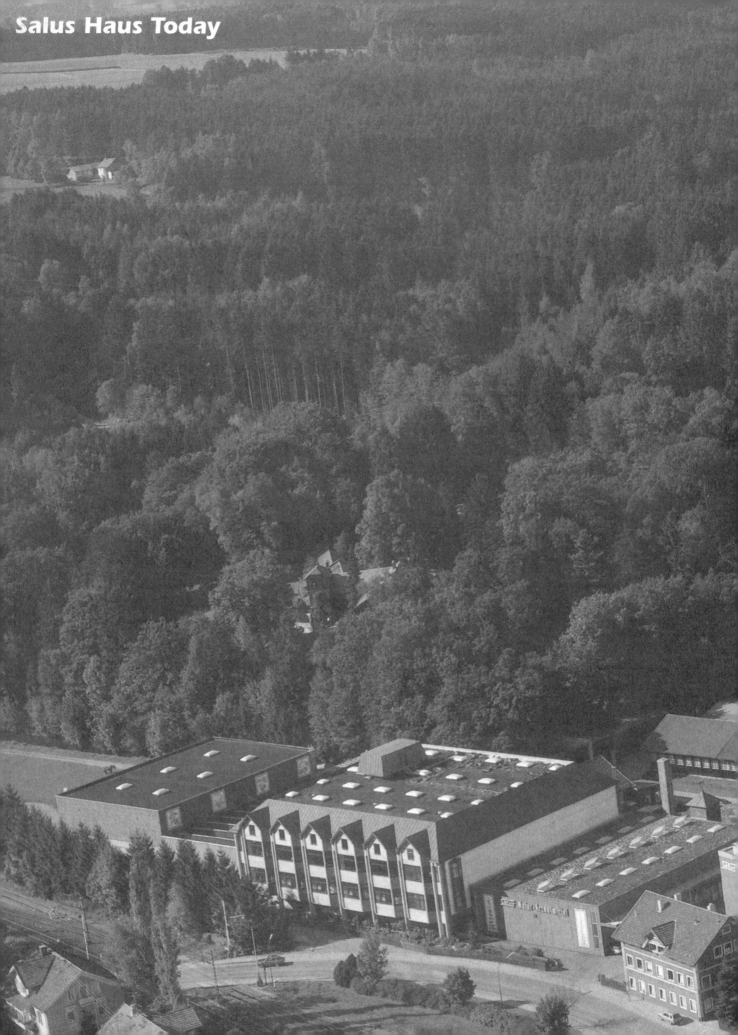
Salus Haus Today

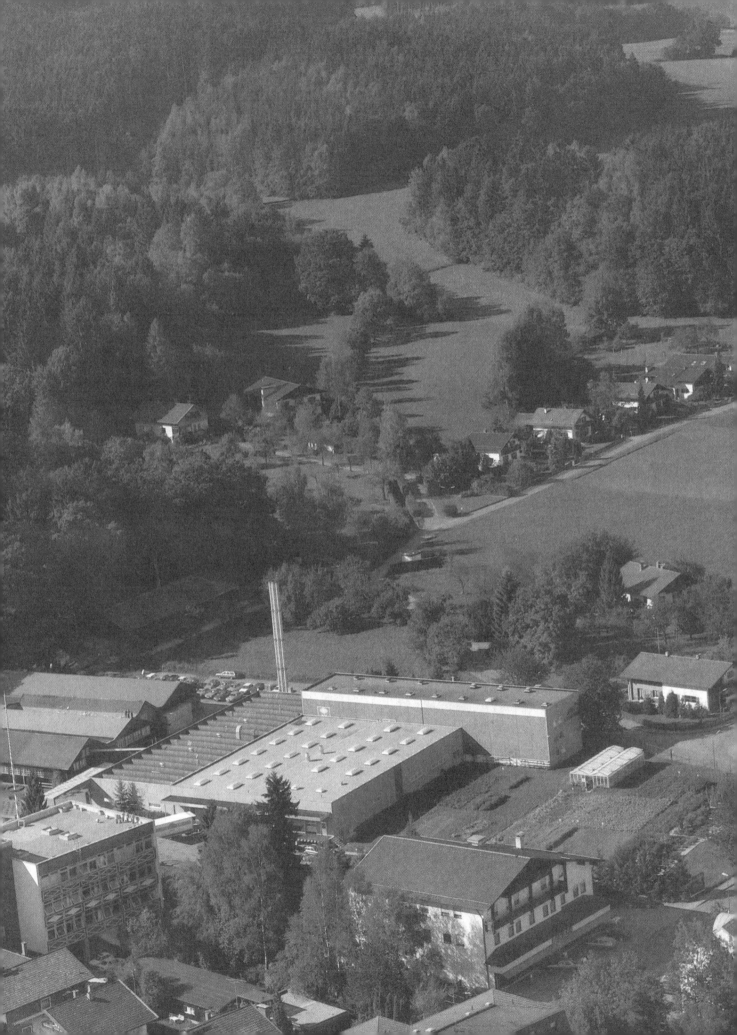

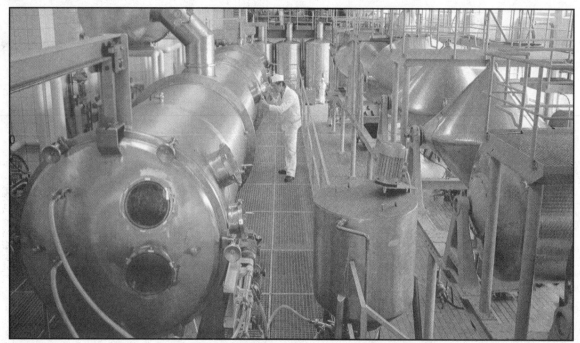

Salus Haus Manufacture of dry extracts of herbs, using Vacuum Drying Tunnel.

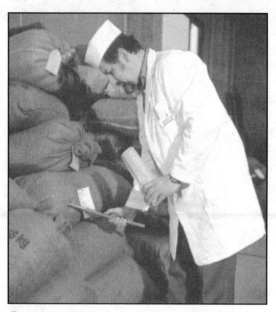

Raw materials being sampled at Salus Haus.

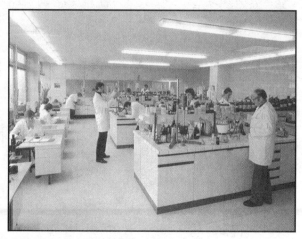

Salus Haus Laboratory.

Salus Haus but, naturally, related; and each company distributes the others' products. Cooperation is close and ongoing. One of these three companies is Flora, headed by Thomas Greither.

The headquarters of the Canadian company, Flora, is located on the banks of the mighty Fraser river, in a suburb of Vancouver B.C. called Burnaby. It's a stunningly beautiful area, situated on the edge of the great Canadian wilderness. The air is crystal clear, and the waters in the surrounding rivers, lakes, and streams are virtually unpolluted, providing the perfect environment for a company in the business of promoting "super health." The original purpose of Dr. Otto Greither in forming Salus house, "to produce the highest quality natural products to cleanse and purify the body," has perhaps found it's ultimate expression in Flora.

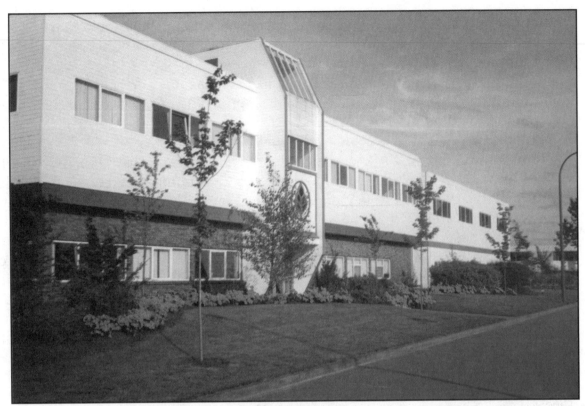

Flora Manufacturing and Distributing, International Headquarters, Burnaby, British Columbia, Canada.

But that should come as no surprise. The importance and responsibility to continue to improve upon the legacy bequeathed to him by both his father and grandfather was instilled in Thomas Greither from the time he was born. That responsibility has become the guiding purpose of Thomas Greither's life. To appreciate the evolution of the Greither legacy at Flora under the leadership of Thomas Greither we have included Flora's mission statement which is provided to their customers and their employees:

IN GOD WE TRUST

The Mission of Flora Distributors is to participate in the continuing evolution of the people of earth towards universal harmony, peace and perfection by providing products and services for the purification and upliftment of the body and the spirit, and by providing each person who derives a livelihood from Flora with an opportunity for personal growth and advancement of these goals in life.

An associate of Elaine's put her in touch with Thomas Greither and they had their first meeting in May, 1992. The meeting was fated. As in the first encounter between Rene and Dr. Brusch, and the subsequent meeting years later between Dr. Brusch and Elaine, there was an instant communion of souls with Elaine and Thomas, perhaps an unspoken understanding that each of them were on a similar spiritual path.

It could not have been a more auspicious occasion. The central purpose of the Greither dynasty, from the time of its founder Dr. Otto Greither, had been to produce high quality natural products which cleansed and purified the body. What better product to become associated with than Essiac.

What was meant to be a short introduction meeting between Elaine and Thomas turned into four hours of non-stop communication between Elaine, Thomas, and most of the key employees of Flora. Elaine explained the entire story of Essiac in exacting and dramatic detail as only Elaine could. Thomas in turn explained to Elaine what his goals were, and the history of his family.

He took her on a tour of the entire Flora facility. She saw the massive warehouse which housed more than 900 product lines, either manufactured or distributed world wide by Flora. She learned that the raw materials used in Flora's products came from every corner of the globe. Flora looked primarily for medicinal plants growing in their natural habitat or from biological cultivation. It was explained to Elaine that because quality begins with the raw material used, the raw materials are monitored with the strictest quality control standards at Flora. For some of the raw materials quality control starts as early as the cultivation stage. Requested samples are subject to an intensive receiving inspection. Laboratory tests are run for identity and content, and purity. The sample values are then taken as a basis for purchasing decisions. Furthermore, each subsequent delivery of raw materials is compared with the values of the purchase sample in order to be released for further processing.

Once the raw materials have been approved as complying with Flora's laboratory standards of quality, the first stage is cutting and sifting. Elaine saw how the bales of herbs were gently loosened using ultramodern technical equipment, how

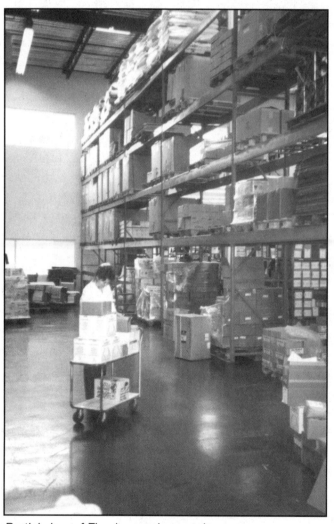

Partial view of Flora's massive warehouse.

initial coarse foreign components were removed by air stream, and how the herbs were cut. The herbs are then weighed and mixed in industrial hygienic mixing drums.

Elaine saw Flora's extraction center and was told that it was the nerve center for the production of all of Flora's fluid preparations. Fluid preparations make up a large portion of Flora's products. They come in a wide range of forms and sizes. Tonics, elixirs, herbal drops and tinctures. Widely differing methods are used for the production of medicinal extracts. Percolation, maceration and distillation. But the purpose they fulfill is the same in each case: to obtain the maximum yield of unadulterated active ingredients using the most gentle extraction methods possible.

She saw the research department and the impressive laboratory facilities. One of the major functions of Flora's state of the art laboratory is not only to produce new products but to monitor Flora's products in every production phase. By the end of the tour Elaine was thoroughly convinced of Flora's ability to do whatever was necessary to finally bring Essiac into the eager hands of suffering humanity. Flora met and exceeded every possible criteria both she and Dr. Brusch had been searching for all these years.

Elaine felt Rene was watching and knew her dream was about to become a reality. Only the details needed to be worked out. As far as Thomas was concerned he was deeply moved by Elaine and her dedication to helping suffering people. He definitely wanted to be involved in producing the Essiac formula on a massive scale, but first of course Thomas would have to investigate Elaine's story further and do his own research on the formulation.

He did just that, and what he discovered was shocking even to a man who had grown up in a family that produced some of the best cleansing products in the world, not to mention his own advanced herbal cleansing products produced at Flora!

Never had he seen an herbal formulation that had such remarkable powers to cleanse and purify the entire system. Trying on himself a sample formulation he had mixed in his own laboratory, he was to experience its immediate effects. Thomas Greither, hardly unhealthy – a strict vegetarian, taking great care in every aspect of his health – could not believe the amount of residual toxins his body seemed to throw off after taking just one treatment of Essiac. The reports from his staff, many of whom had also tried the Essiac formulation, were dramatic to say the least. Everybody at Flora, which is organized like one large family, all sharing in the decision making and profits of the company, was thrilled at the prospect of being involved with the Essiac project.

The only thing that remained was to come up with a suitable name, something that expressed the true spirit of Essiac, but made no cancer curing claims whatsoever. After a lot of thought by the entire Flora team, the name Flor•Essence was chosen. It was decided upon for three reasons: First, the Essiac formula is the *essence* of Dr. Otto Greither's original purpose, to cleanse and purify the body. Second, Dr. Greither's original purpose is today the *essence* of Flora. Third, the *essence* of God's medicinal plants (flora) is to restore radiant health. Flor•Essence is "a holy drink which purifies the body and puts it back in balance with the great spirit." The Ojibwa medicine man would approve. The circle was complete, the holy drink was now hopefully beyond the jealous and suspicious reach of the Medical Establishment and would soon be in the hands of a neglected, suffering humanity, back on the path of balance and purity.

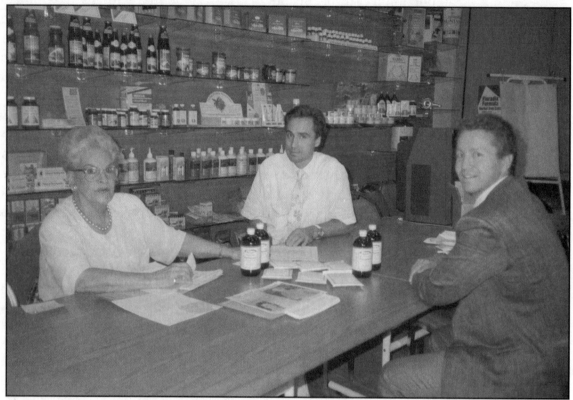

Planning for the future. Elaine Alexander, Thomas Greither (center) Proprietor and Managing Director of Flora, and Dean Parks, Marketing Director, in Flora's conference room.

A short time after Elaine Alexander had met with Flora, *The Vancouver Sun,* British Columbia's leading daily newspaper (part of the powerful Canada-wide Southam chain) came out with an article entitled *Keeping Hope Alive.* Elaine had no idea when the article was coming out, or the size of it when she met Thomas. She was under the impression that some day the paper might do a small story on her involvement with Essiac, and gave it little thought.

As it turned out, the small story became a three page feature article in *The Sun's* 'Saturday Review'. It was a fresh look at the Rene Caisse story with a special focus on Elaine Alexander and her continuing work as the present torch bearer of the Essiac Legacy. It described in some detail how she had become the inheritor of the Essiac formula and what she planned to do in the future. But it failed to give information about her recent partnership with Flora, since most of the research for the article had been done prior to her association with this company.

Once again the story of Essiac awakened the public. The response was overwhelming. People called Elaine incessantly, so much so that she had to have new lines installed in her house to keep up with the incoming traffic. Other people found out where she lived. A steady flow of suffering individuals arrived at all hours of the day and night seeking her help and advice. And once again she heard horrendous stories of pain and suffering. But this time Elaine had more than just advice and consolation to give. She was finally able to tell her fellow human beings that Essiac would soon be available for anyone who desired it. Obtaining it was as simple as walking into their local health food store and asking for it. Its new name was Flor•Essence.

Rene's dream was a reality.

━━━━━◆━━━━━

Flor•Essence can now be purchased in nearly every health food store in Canada and some in the United States. If it is not availabe in your local health food store Flor•Essence can be purchased by simply writing or calling the following mail order distributors:

P.A.H. Products
P.O. Box 2665
Mission, KS 66201
1-800-318-2666

Swanson Products
P.O. Box 2803
Fargo, ND 58102
1-701-277-1662

L & H Vitamins
37-10 Crescent St.
Long Island City, NY 11101
1-718-937-7400

Flor•Essence is produced in both ready-to-take liquid form and formulated dry herbs which can be easily brewed at home. The distribution of Flor•Essence in the United States will be expanding in the near future. Flor•Essence is sold simply as an herbal cleansing tea. No claims are made. But as envisioned, word has begun to spread. We have included in the Appendix some testimonials provided by terminal cancer patients who have used Flor•Essence and have achieved remarkable results.

(At this writing, A prostate/urinary tract herbal formula will soon be available. It has been used with great success through the years and is also known to enhance the cleansing action – discharge of toxins – of Flor•Essence.)

Section Three will provide more details about the formula.

Section Three

Flor•Essence
The Formula

"There are more things in heaven and earth, Horatio, than are dreamt of in your philosophy."

Hamlet
William Shakespeare

The Grand Medicine Society

To begin to understand the *essence* of Flor•Essence it is important to remember and appreciate its true originators, the proud Ojibwa.

At the turn of the century in northern Ontario, the Ojibwa still lived as they had for thousands of years, supremely in touch with nature, guided by their visions, trusting completely in their ancient traditions. The Ojibwa

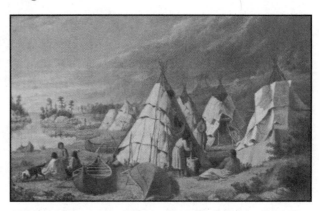

Typical 19th century Ojibwa village. Painting by Paul Kane.

medicine man, who gave his remarkable herbal healing brew (the brew which eventually evolved into Flor•Essence) to the English woman stricken with breast cancer, was most assuredly a member of the *Midewiwan* – The Grand Medicine Society of the Ojibwa, a venerated group of men and women skilled in the arts of healing. Their knowledge of both herbal healing cures and the *Manitous* – supernatural powers – was second to none throughout all of native America.

According to Basil Johnston (himself an Ojibwa, author of *Ojibwa Heritage* and linguist and lecturer at the department of Ethology, Royal Ontario Museum in Toronto) the path to membership in the *Midewiwan* was long and arduous:

"The aspirant, who must be selected for membership by a *Mide* (medicine man) had first to serve an apprenticeship, paying a Mide master for instruction in the secrets of herbal cures, and in the myths and rituals that evoked the *Manitous* powers. Then came an elaborate multiday initiation rite that tested the novice's abilities. Only thereafter was he or she permitted to practice the healing arts. This first initiation was only a beginning. There were four ranks of *Mides*, the highest of which required four separate apprenticeships and four initiations, each demanding more than the previous one. Few attained this eminence, and those who did were regarded with special awe, as they were endowed with enormous healing knowledge. To have attained the fourth rank could take the better part of a life time."

The Ojibwa believed that all plants possessed an incorporeal being, a unique soul-spirit, a vitalizing substance that gave to its physical form, growth and healing powers. In addition, plants had a more wonderful power, the power to conjoin with other plants to form a unified spirit, many times stronger than the spirit of a single plant. It was this "unified" spirit which endowed their herbal medications with such tremendous healing power.

Before the plants were picked, usually in the late summer, the *Mides* would say a prayer:

Your spirit,
my spirit,
may they unite to make
one spirit in healing,
you have given beauty,
now we ask that you give
the gift of well being.

How the *Mides* knew which plants to pick for specific illnesses was learned from several sources. Knowledge came in the form of visions, contact with the spirit world, intuition, and observation. For thousands of years the Ojibwa had observed the behavior of animals when ill or injured, in particular which plants these animals would consume to heal themselves. From their astute observations, their visions, their guidance from the Grand Fathers, and their own intuition, they amassed a wealth of knowledge, passing it down from generation to generation.

They, of course, tested numerous variations of their remedies, until they found the very best possible cures for every affliction experienced by their people. For the Ojibwa, disease was caused by impurities in the body and spirit. An impure condition put one out of balance with the Great Spirit who informed all things in the world. Healing was a process of purification of both the body and the soul. The cures used by the Mides, herbal and ritual, were always directed towards purification in order to put one back in balance with the Great Spirit. It is therefore not surprising that when the old Ojibwa medicine man gave his healing brew to the English woman dying of breast cancer he told her that it was "a holy drink that would purify her body and place her back in balance with the great spirit."

Midewiwan literally translates to *good hearted*. To be an Ojibwa medicine man, you had to be *good hearted*. What better way to express your good heart than to help suffering people. We owe a great deal of gratitude to the Ojibwa and their sacred knowledge of the healing power of plants. Without their sacred knowledge and their *good heart* to pass it on, there would be no Flor•Essence.

Plant Power

There is ample precedent to view herbs as potent healers. In fact the history of medicine is largely the history of the healing properties discovered in plants. According to a documentary entitled "The Hidden Power of Plants," presented by PBS:

> "Around the world, traditional healers today, using plant medications, provide health care to eighty percent of the human population, over four billion people. Over 25 percent of the drugs prescribed in the U.S. contain plant materials as their principal active ingredients."

Childhood leukemia and other cancers have been treated since the 1950's with vincristne, an alkaloid which comes from periwinkle, an evergreen plant. Digitalis, an important heart medication, comes from the leaves of the foxglove plant. Penicillin comes from a mold, and is therefore plant based. Many other antibiotics are based on substances produced by fungi.

But long before science discovered the healing power of plants or even believed that they existed, so-called "primitive" people were healing themselves with *God's Pharmacy.*

South American Indians for centuries have been treating fevers, especially malarial fevers, with a special tea made from bark of the Cinchona tree. Scientist were later to discover that Cinchona bark is a potent source of Quinine.

American Indians for centuries have been treating a multitude of aches and pains with an herbal brew made from white willow bark. Today synthesized and refined willow bark, acetylsalicylic acid, is known to us as Aspirin!

Natural healers from around the world have used over 3,000 plant species in the treatment of cancer alone! There is an abundance of scientific literature on plants and herbs which cite their anticancer effects in lab studies, clinical tests, and human experiences.

However, the Medical Establishment does not use plants for healing in the same manner as natural healers. Now that the drug companies have realized that some plants do in fact possess healing powers, they have naturally figured out a method to capitalize on those powers in a big way.

Vast amounts of resources are expended by the major pharmaceutical companies in order to isolate a bioactive compound from a medicinal plant, and then to make some molecular modifications to it; that way, their synthetic product can become *exclusive* or proprietary. Then they can recoup the 125 million or so that it costs to test a new drug and bring it to market.

Synthetic pills usually only contain an isolated chemical compound. Pharmaceutical scientists will take one chemical from a plant, leaving behind hundreds of other compounds, plus all the minerals, vitamins, and fibers that accompany this one chemical in the live plant.

But there is a big problem with this approach, notes Dr. Laurence Badgley, M.D.

> "Each raw herb has a unique combination of chemicals in it. An herb's medicinal effect is the result of the synergistic activity, the working together of all the chemicals that the herb contains. By ingesting a synthetic *chemical isolate* whose molecular chains have been altered in the laboratory we may be depriving ourselves of the herb's full healing powers."

The Essence of Flor▪Essence

Flor•Essence contains only certified whole *organic* raw herbs, all harvested at the proper time to insure potency, and all dried using a special water

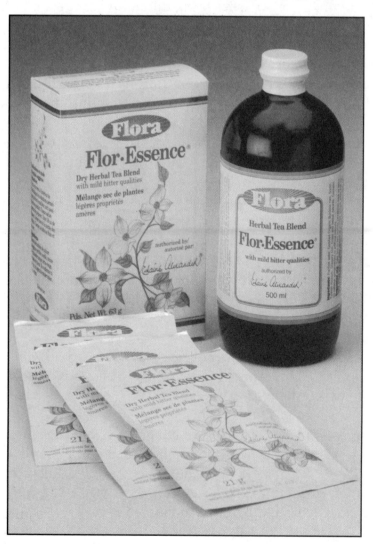

extraction process to further guarantee maximum effectiveness. The core of the Flor•Essence formula, passed on by the Ojibwa medicine man, is sheep sorrel, burdock root, slippery elm, and rhubarb root.

As was mentioned in Section One, Dr. Brusch added other herbs to the *core* formula when he found that the additional herbs (usually imported and thus unavailable to the Ojibwa) worked as powerful *potentiators* to the core formula. The formula which is now called Flor• Essence has in fact been proven by Dr. Brusch to be even more effective than the original formula, but it should be emphasized that the core of the formula passed on by the Ojibwa medicine man has been retained in Flor•Essence... its heart and soul.

The proportions among the herbs contained in Flor•Essence remains a closely guarded secret. Simply knowing which herbs are in the formula won't do. The key is the proportion. It has got to be right.

The Ojibwa believed the most important aspect of their herbal healing medications was the relationship among the different plants used within a particular medication. They had to be in balance, in harmony, to act as one unified healing spirit. We have another word for unified spirit, that word is *synchronous*. Any attempt to explain the healing power of Flor•Essence by describing the healing properties known to exist within each individual herb contained in Flor•Essence, will only serve as a partial explanation of the true healing miracle of Flor•Essence. The whole of Flor•Essence is definitely much more than the sum of its parts.

Why and how Flor•Essence ultimately works may never be fully understood. But to someone who has recovered from terminal cancer by using the formula, it usually doesn't matter.

However, even though it is impossible to completely explain how Flor•Essence bestows its gifts, we will now briefly describe some of what is known about the remarkable core healing herbs in Flor•Essence:

SHEEP SORREL – Rene Caisse felt this herb was the most active cancer fighter among all the herbs present in the old Indian brew. "The herb that will destroy cancer... is the dog-eared sheep sorrel, sometimes called sour grass," she

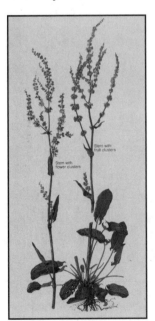

said on a number of occasions. And she may have been right. Interestingly, for hundreds of years sheep sorrel has appeared in historical archives in both America and Europe as a remedy for cancer. In 1926, the National Cancer Institute was presented with a recipe from Canada which was said to be an old Indian cure for cancer. The main ingredient was none other than sheep sorrel.

Rene Caisse observed that not only was sheep sorrel effective in attacking and breaking down tumors, it also was effective in alleviating many chronic conditions and degenerative diseases.

It has been reported by other researchers that sheep sorrel relieves internal ulcers, black jaundice and virtually all skin diseases.

The seeds of sheep sorrel steeped in wine have been used to stop hemorrhages and heavy menstrual flow. In addition the seeds contain an anitivenomous property that relieves bites and rids the body of poisons.

Sheep sorrel reportedly acts as a tonic for the urinary tract. Poultices can be made with an infusion of the leaves and applied directly to boils and tumors. In 1475, Thorleif Bjornsson, author of an Iceland Medical Manuscript, wrote, "Its juice put in the eyes makes them bright... its juice in the ear makes one hear well.

If one wears it a scorpion will not hurt him." *(We are not however recommending it as a scorpion repellent.)*

Sheep sorrel contains high amounts of vitamins A & B-complex, especially in its seed, C, D, E, K, P and vitamin U. It's also rich in minerals, including calcium, chlorine, iron, magnesium, silicon, sodium, sulphur, and trace amounts of copper, iodine, manganese, and zinc.

Other vital health-giving elements in sheep sorrel are the carotenoids and *chlorophyll* which are present in the leaves and stems, and several organic acids which include malic, oxalic, tannic, tartaric, and citric, an antioxidant.

Chlorophyll, the substance which makes plants green, resembles hemoglobin in human blood. And like hemoglobin carries oxygen to every cell in your body.

It has been reported that chlorophyll:

- Inhibits chromosome damage and this action may effectively block cancer.
- Increases your resistance to X rays.
- Eliminates germs and inhibits the growth of harmful bacteria.
- Reduces the damaging effects of radiation burns.
- Stimulates the regeneration of fresh tissue.
- Purifies the liver and relieves pancreas inflammation.
- Dramatically raises the oxygen level in the tissue cells.
- Cleanses the walls of blood vessels.
- Strengthens the cell walls, which may improve the function of the heart, intestines, lungs, uterus, and vascular system.

To increase oxygen at the cellular level may be vital in eliminating cancer. Otto Warbur in the 1930's demonstrated that cancer cannot grow rapidly in the presence of oxygen. His theory was that cancer is a process of cell mutation engendered by a lack of oxygen at the cellular level. He reasoned that any effective cancer therapy must increase the oxygen content of the blood. Because chlorophyll increases the oxygen content of the blood, it may in fact decrease cell mutation and therefore counteract cancer. Chlorophyll, also because of its high oxygen content, may be effective against other conditions including AIDS and HIV-related viruses.

Research at the Linus Pauling Institute and the Anderson Hospital in Texas has shown that chlorophyll juice produces some immunity against many carcinogens and strengthens the immune system. Japanese researchers have reportedly discovered that chlorophyll juice inhibits chromosome damage, which is a precursor to cancer.

Carotenoid is a vital element in chlorophyll. Hungarian researchers have found that the leaves of sheep sorrel have a total carotenoid content of 8-12 percent.

Beta carotene is a member of the family of carotenoids. Research from multiple sources has shown that beta carotene is converted to vitamin A in our liver. Vitamin A strengthens the immune system by increasing the production of white blood cells. It is white blood cells that destroy cancer cells. Beta carotene is an antioxidant which means it can control the build-up of harmful free radicals. Free radicals can actually alter genes and seriously damage cell walls.

All carotenoids and especially beta carotene are coming under closer scientific scrutiny because of their ability to strengthen the immune system. Dr. Harinder Garewal at the University of Arizona Cancer Center in Tucson found that precancerous lesions in the mouth diminished in size in 70% of the patients tested with only 30 mg of carotene a day.

Sheep sorrel is rich in oxalic acid in the form of potassium oxalate. Oxalic acid has been shown to be a powerful oxidizing acid which stimulates the human system into activity. Oxalic acid combines with calcium to aid in digestive assimilation, plus oxalic acid stimulates the peristaltic action of the intestines and may even be responsible for increased blood coagulation. Using just the root of the sheep sorrel people have gained improvement from stomach hemorrhages and jaundice conditions.

It can be seen then that sheep sorrel, a truly remarkable herb by itself, surely plays a vital role as part of the great healing power of Flor•Essence.

BURDOCK ROOT – It has been known for centuries to natural healers throughout the world as a powerful blood purifier. In the last half of the twentieth century burdock root has attracted the attention of cancer researchers in both Hungary and Japan. In 1966 two Hungarian scientists reported "considerable anti-tumor activity" in purified fraction of burdock. And in 1984 Japanese scientists working at Nagoya university discovered a substance in burdock root capable of

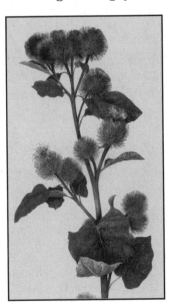

reducing cell mutation, either in the absence or in the presence of metabolic activation. So important is this new property that Japanese researchers named it "the B-factor," for burdock factor.

As a blood purifier burdock root may clear congestion in circulatory, lymphatic, respiratory and urinary systems. It can help eliminate excess fluids in the body and stimulate the elimination of toxic waste materials which will relieve liver disorders and improve digestion. It can cleanse the body of bile, detoxify the kidneys and gall bladder. Burdock root can increase perspiration which in turn carries off excess toxins.

The Chinese consider burdock root an excellent rejuvenator and aphrodisiac. Burdock root has been used as a diuretic to relieve infectious diseases, especially those of the urinary-genital tract, and also to treat arthritis, rheumatism and sciatica.

Burdock root is rich in vitamins, B-complex, E, and P. It also contains, in high amounts, chromium, cobalt, iron magnesium, phosphorus, silicon zinc, sodium and potassium.

The root is composed mostly of carbohydrates, largely inulin (*not* insulin!) some mucilage and starches, and some sugar.

Inulin, the principle ingredient in burdock root, has been shown to have remarkable curative powers. Inulin helps strengthen the organs and its natural sugar content helps regulate blood sugar metabolism. (In fact Flor•Essence has been shown to eliminate the need for insulin in diabetics.) The inulin in burdock root probably plays a key role in clearing up diabetic conditions, because of its ability to regulate sugar metabolism.

Inulin reportedly is a powerful immune modulator because it is said to hook onto the surface of white blood cells and make them work better.

In animal experiments, burdock root extracts have been shown to destroy bacteria and fungus cultures, as well as showing strong anti-tumor activity. Burdock root, the second wonder herb in Flor•Essence.

SLIPPERY ELM BARK – One of the world's best known herbal remedies. The principle component of slippery elm bark is mucilage. Mucilage is a naturally formed viscous or sticky fiber which consists of a gum dissolved in the juices of a plant. The mucilage in slippery elm bark is similar to that found in flax seed.

Slippery elm bark is one of nature's miracle cleansers. Its sticky substance dissolves mucus that has been deposited in organ tissue, lymph glands and nerve chan-

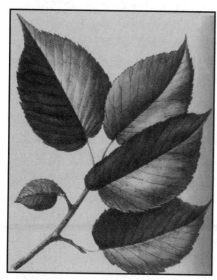

nels. Its lubricating action protects and softens all the membrane linings in the body, especially damaged and inflamed areas. It buffers the effects of increased discharge of urine through the urinary tract. (Increased urine usually occurs as a result of the detoxifying abilities of some of the other herbs included in the Flor•Essence formula.)

Slippery elm bark's sticky adhesive quality also lubricates the bones and joints, gathers up dissolved toxic waste material from all areas in the body including the bowel and then helps to discharge them. As the mucilaginous material passes through the alimentary canal, it coats the organs over which it flows with a sticky film. This action reduces irritation, reduces sensitivity to acids and bitters and most importantly slows down the entry of harmful chemicals. Slippery elm bark can help reduce the pain of ulcers and eventually heal them by restoring normal mucous coating to irritated tissues.

When applied externally, slippery elm bark has been shown to have extraordinary healing properties. The mucilage penetrates wounds and covers them. Impurities are drawn out of abrasions, abscesses or ulcers. Slippery elm bark reportedly has the ability to grow new cells to repair tissues. The new cells form fresh skin which readily forms over sores and quickens the healing process.

It has been reported that tumors are reduced in female organs when a suppository made with water and a powder made from slippery elm bark is used. Inflammation of the vagina and uterus have been relieved with a douche consisting of a decoction of the bark. Slippery elm bark also produces an antibiotic and antimicrobial effect.

Slippery elm bark like all the herbs in Flor•Essence is rich in both vitamins and minerals.

RHUBARB ROOT – Another remarkable detoxifying herb which has also been used throughout the world for centuries because of its proven healing properties. As early as 220 B.C. the Chinese were using rhubarb root as a medicine because they believed it to eliminate excess heat from the small intestines. Excess heat in the small intestines was an indication (according to Chinese medicine) of toxins in the blood, which they felt was responsible for many diseases.

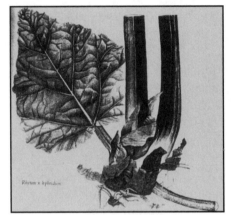

Rhubarb root purges the body of bile, parasites, and stagnating food by stimulating the gall duct to expel toxic waste matter. It has been shown to alleviate chronic liver problems by cleansing the liver.

Rhubarb root has been shown to improve digestion and increase the appetite. It has also been shown to help heal ulcers, alleviate disorders of the spleen and colon, relieve constipation, and help heal hemorrhoids and bleeding in the upper digestive tract.

Studies in the 1980's have shown rhubarb root extract to contain antibiotic, antimicrobial and antitumor properties. Rhubarb root, in addition to having concentrated amounts of both vitamins and minerals, contains a remarkable substance called rhein. Recent studies at the Oriental Medicine Research Center in Tokyo, Japan, indicate rhein inhibits the growth of pathogenic bacteria in the intestines. It is believed that rhein is also effective against Candida albicans, fever and inflammation, as well as pain.

This information barely begins to touch on the healing possibilities of the individual *core* herbs in Flor•Essence, nor does it describe the additional healing properties of the vital *potentiating* herbs: *Watercress, blessed thistle, red clover, and kelp.* Any good herbal reference manual can give you a more complete picture of the remarkable healing properties existing within the *core* herbs and the additional *potentiating* herbs.

However, once again, it should be emphasized that the true healing power of Flor•Essence is derived from the synchronous effect (the "unified spirit') of the *entire* formula, not from the sum of the *individual* healing properties existing within the herbs present in Flor•Essence.

It is the benefits derived from the entire formula that we will now address.

Here is a compilation and a paraphrase of some of what Rene Caisse had to say about the *old* Indian brew:

"My treatment is non-toxic herbs. It goes to the seat of the trouble no matter where it is whether internal or on the surface, and gives healthy cells the strength to resist the demands of the malignant cells for the substance upon which the malignancy thrives, thus causing a recession of the malignant cells from the healthy cells, which have become stronger.

I can truthfully say that I have in many cases been able to stay the disease (cancer) and in some really bad cases prolong life. In practically all cases, pain and suffering were alleviated so that the patient was not compelled to resort to opiates or narcotics in increasing doses, as usually is the case. My decoction is a non-toxic drink made from herbs which are of definite benefit for cancer.

I have felt that once the cancer becomes active, travelling as it does along the line of least resistance...insidiously, on its relentless course, any destructive agency applied to the human body can only do more harm (chemotherapy, radiation, surgery).

I have found that no matter where the malignancy may be in the human body, surgery would be much more successful after treatment with my herbal remedy, followed by continued treatment over a period of time; then there would be no recurrence of the tumor. In the case of breast cancer, the primary growth will usually invade the mammary gland of the opposite breast or the auxilla (armpit), or both. My treatment, I found, reduces the secondary growth into the primary mass, enlarging it for a time. When it became localized, it was encapsulated and could then be removed without danger of recurrence. *In one instance, a patient with breast cancer was instructed by her doctor to take my treatment before undergoing surgery, however after a brief treatment the cancer had completely disappeared, with no recurrence.*

Most importantly, and this was verified in animal tests conducted at the Brusch Medical Center and other laboratories, it was discovered that one of the most dramatic effects of taking this remedy was *its affinity for drawing all the cancer cells, which had spread, back to the original site, at which point the tumor would first harden, then later it would soften, until it vanished altogether* or, more realistically, the tumor would decrease in size to where it could then be surgically removed with minimal complications.

In certain cases and at certain stages of the disease, the cancer would act as if it were 'coming to a head,' similar to an abscess. It would then break down and slough away. These people *all reported that when the mass breaks, it isn't like puss but like a cottage cheese substance that comes away. Still other types will enlarge until the mass is localized, then loosen and reduce in size until there is nothing left, having been absorbed into and carried off by the blood stream and body waste.*

Other observations I've made over my years of practice: The treatment allowed patients to sleep in greater comfort than they had in the past, and the increased appetite and weight, diminished pain, decreased tumor size and longer life span were all attested to by doctors in attendance. Dr. Banting, who examined case after case, was especially impressed with the effect of the treatment on the pancreas and possibly other sluggish glands which it seemed to restore to activity. Other doctors who examined my patients discovered the treatment had a special effect on the liver. After taking blood counts they found hemoglobin and white cell platelets had returned to normal.

My treatment, given to people in health, is helpful in that it is a blood purifier and will do its work before there is any chance of the malignant cells invading the body."

During one of the radio interviews between Elaine Alexander and Dr. Brusch, Elaine asked Dr. Brush if he knew of other diseases or serious health problems the old Indian healing brew might benefit. Dr. Brusch's answer was brief and to the point:

"It will greatly improve any condition afflicting the body. "

Quite a remarkable claim, but one that is not without living proof, anecdotal as it may well be. (See Testimonials in the Appendix.)

The Ultimate Detoxifier

There is universal agreement among natural healers both past and present that detoxifying your body is probably the single most important thing you can do to restore or maintain good health. Detoxification, (purification) is the central unifying theme behind the entire story of this remarkable herbal treatment. All of the major players from the Ojibwa to Flora have realized that purification is the key to healing and a long life of radiant health.

Most cleansing agents are used over a fairly short period of time. In addition most cleansing agents have some unpleasant side effects, usually headache and nausea, for example.

Flor•Essence is much different. It can be taken safely over a long period of time (for an active illness) with nothing but beneficial results. For use as a preventative or tonic if wished, a shorter *or* longer period of use is perfectly safe. There are no side effects and it can be taken along with any other therapies, orthodox or otherwise.

Dr. Brusch felt the formula actually had the ability to identify particular toxins, gather them up, break them down, and then discharge them.

A detoxified system strengthens the immune system, which may in part be why Flor•Essence is believed to be so effective; not only against cancer but against a multiplicity of other diseases which include:

Hypoglycemia

Multiple sclerosis

Parkinson's

Arthritis

Chronic Fatigue Syndrome

Ulcers

Thyroid problems

Fibroids

Hemorrhoids

Prostate and urinary problems

Circulation

Diabetes

Malignancies

Sleeping disorders

Warts

Psoriasis

Impotence

Alzheimer's

Asthma

And allergies.

Is there clinical evidence to support this? No, but as stated, there are numerous certified testimonies which are quite convincing. (See the Appendix.)

Other potential benefits of Flor•Essence are:

1. Calms the body, because it is a natural sedative.
2. Decreases pain and can eliminate it altogether in many severe cases.
3. Stops hemmorages, yet builds up the blood.
4. Prevents or corrects constipation.
5. Restores taste buds.
6. Helps digestion.
7. Cures insomnia.
8. Boosts immune system (of great benefit while undergoing radical cancer therapies).
9. Works as a wonderful preventative tonic.
10. Helps heal intestinal burns from radiation therapy.
11. Helps prevent the detrimental effect of aluminum, lead, and mercury poisoning.
12. Reduces heavy metal deposits in tissue, especially those surrounding the joints. Relieves inflammation and stiffness. This may be why Flor•Essence works against arthritic symptoms.
13. Protects against toxins entering the brain.
14. Instills a feeling of overall well being.
15. Decreases nodular mass.

However a word of caution is in order:

The action of Flor•Essence to localize growths within the body and then to break them down and flush them out along with all poisons and toxins is truly a wonderful thing. But too much of a good thing can be dangerous. If you exceed the recommended dosage of Flor•Essence you could be at risk, because broken down materials may be expelled too rapidly from your body, causing some of the materials to form a blockage. We know of no case of this happening but it is a theoretical possibility. Therefore it is highly recommended that you follow the daily recommended dosage of Flor•Essence prescribed by Flora.

The following information is offered by Flora to prospective users of Flor•Essence:

What you should know about Flor•Essence

The whole purpose in starting on this wonderful old therapy is, of course, to obtain the greatest benefit from it. This being so, certain important factors should be known by those who take it. Natural therapies take time to re-awaken the healing process and restore health to something that's taken a long time to develop, so be patient!

Overall, Rene Caisse's patients took her treatment on the longer rather than the shorter term, often a year or more. Certainly until proof of stable improvement was shown. The total daily dosage was gradually decreased until a maintenance dosage (2 oz once a day) was reached. This smaller amount could be continued as long as desired.

Suggested Use

Preventative or Tonic:
- Shake the Flor•Essence liquid well before use.
- Measure out 1 to 2 oz (28-56 ml) once daily.
- Dilute with an equal or double amount of unfluoridated, boiled hot water.
- Sip slowly.
- For best results, take on an empty stomach either a.m. or p.m, prior to retiring.

Extra Strength (For Active Illness):
- Measure out 2 oz (56 ml) once or twice daily.
- Dilute with an equal or double amount of unfluoridated, boiled hot water.
- Sip slowly.
- Take on an empty stomach, in p.m. prior to retiring and in a.m. 1 hour before breakfast.

Maximum Strength:
- Measure out 2 oz (56 ml) three times daily. Dilute with equal or double amount of unfluoridated, boiled, hot water.
- Sip slowly. When improvement stable, cut back to twice daily.

For Children:
• Maximum daily amount 1 1/2 oz to 2 oz (42-56 ml).
• Dilute with equal or double amount of unfluoridated, boiled hot water.
• Sip slowly. Give on empty stomach, half the daily amount in p.m. prior to retiring and half the daily amount in a.m. one hour before breakfast.
• Keep out of their reach.

For Infants:
• Maximum daily amount 1 oz (28 ml).
• Dilute with equal or double amount of unfluoridated, boiled hot water.
• Sip slowly. Give on empty stomach, half the daily amount in p.m. prior to retiring and half the daily amount in a.m. When suitable.
• Keep out of their reach.

SIP THE TEA. TAKE 3 OR 4 MINUTES TO DRINK IT.

* Note: Flor•Essence comes in two forms. Already brewed liquid and pre-mixed dry herbs. The simple directions for preparing the dry herbal tea blend comes with the package.

The herbs used in Flor•Essence contain no pesticides, insecticides, or herbicides, and they are not irradiated. This product will not be identical each time you brew it. This is a natural product, not a "clone" such as the processed assembly line products of which we see so much.

Slippery elm, burdock root and to some degree sheep sorrel all have slippery, glutinous properties. Therefore from time to time (as herbs vary as to colour, look, taste and even smell, depending on the source, when harvested, and the quality), there may be a thickening of the liquid. If this occurs, follow the directions, bottle as is and take the dosage from your bottled liquid (thick or thin). If thick, add more freshly boiled hot water to the concoction. It will then become more liquid, but you will still be taking the same dosage. All the properties needed are contained within, whether you take it one way or the other.

The RESIDUE is not harmful and almost impossible to eliminate when bottling. Some will settle in your bottles, either leave it to settle and take your dosage from the clear liquid, or shake the bottle and take it all.

The RESIDUE is FIBRE (all the properties obtained in the cooking and steeping are in the liquid) but fibre can improve elimination and thus further discharge the build-up of toxins in the body.

Do NOT put the dry herbs in the refrigerator. Keep them in a HEAVY BROWN PAPER BAG (or the package you purchased them in), tightly closed, in a COOL DRY cupboard.

There is something to remember while taking Flor•Essence: it is NOT an ANTIBIOTIC, so have PATIENCE and PERSEVERE! Give it time to do the thorough job it is capable of doing, and it will "re-educate the body," as Dr. Brusch was fond of saying.

We hope this section has given you some idea about the remarkable healing benefits of Flor•Essence. But it would be a mistake to think of Flor•Essence only as something to take when you are suffering from cancer or other serious health problems. Flor•Essence is probably the best preventative tonic on the market today. The optimum time to take Flor•Essence is before you experience the effects of a serious disease.

Many people who are not ill take Flor•Essence to maintain their good health. They report, after taking Flor•Essence for only a short time, a sense of well being they never thought possible: colds disappear, flus are unable to get much of a grip, energy levels soar, and an overall feeling of "super wellness" pervades their entire being. People who have used it to clear up serious diseases report once they recover and continue taking Flor•Essence, they never again experience ill health.

Again, we've only touched on a very small amount of what is known both about the core herbs in Flor•Essence and the benefits of the entire formula as a healer and as a preventative tonic. Its effects are different for everybody who tries it. One of the wonders of the formula is it seems to adapt itself to whatever the problem is.

There are now (and will be in the future) many theories as to why the formula heals. We think the Ojibwa understood its healing miracle best:

"A holy drink that purifies the body and places it back in balance with the great spirit."

Nothing we have said (or for that matter anyone else) could ever describe Flor•Essence's healing action and benefits more profoundly.

Epilogue

It has been said that all great dramas never end, they're simply replayed with new heros and villains. The story of Essiac is no exception. The drama continues.

Flor•Essence, with virtually no advertising, is blossoming. Thousands of people have found their way once again to the old Indian brew. Many of them, given up on by the medical establishment (their doctors having assured them, after consulting their diagnostic crystal balls, that they have only a short time left) have made miraculous recoveries, enough so as to give even the most desperately ill a great deal of hope.

However, as this manuscript goes to press a new wave of oppression has been unleashed by the enforcement wing of the Medical Establishment, the FDA. This time the attack is not directed solely at Flor•Essence, as in the era of Saint Rene, but rather at the entire alternative health care industry.

Under the auspices of consumer protection the FDA has a new, highly aggressive agenda. It is as follows:

1. Make high-potency vitamins (such as vitamin C in excess of 100 mg!), *herbs,* amino acids, and other supplements prescription items only.

2. Prevent dissemination of truthful claims about natural therapies.

The FDA *says* it now wants to regulate herbs and vitamins because of the unsubstantiated potential health claims sometimes made by the manufactures and distributors. The FDA *says* they fear these claims may raise false hopes – as if giving someone hope, false or otherwise, qualifies as a crime. The FDA also *says* that they are deeply concerned about *possible* side effects of high potency vitamins and herbs. This, in spite of the fact that there has not been a single reported death attributed to vitamin or herbal overdose in a decade, possibly never! There is something beyond insanity in all of this when you think of the side effects of chemotherapy and other treatment modalities currently accepted and supported by the FDA. A short stroll through the Physicians Desk Reference (PDR) is enough to make anyone think twice about taking the most commonly prescribed drugs.

What is the *real* reason the FDA is working so hard to limit your access to supplements, *herbs* and vitamins. The FDA has admitted in print that "they do not want the presence of dietary supplements in the market to act as a disincentive to the development of drugs." And therein lies an important clue as to what's going on.

The health food – alternative therapy – industry has grown exponentially in the last decade. So large in fact that it has finally reached mainstream America. In a recent poll over 50 percent of the public said they would consider alternative therapies as an adjunct or *outright choice* over orthodox medicine. And a like number of people have further admitted that they no longer have faith in the therapies employed by their own family doctors.

There has been an enormous shift in public awareness of health issues. The Medical Establishment is keenly aware of this fact. But instead of looking inward to try and determine why they are failing to capture the confidence of the public, instead of recognizing and expediting research to uncover the potentially huge contributions of nutritional supplements, they have chosen to adopt a loser's profile: *Don't fix YOURSELF, kill the competition and then control their market.*

But this time their task will not be as easy as it was in the past.

What we are witnessing today is similar, but not the same, as the public outcry to support Rene Caisse. To be sure she had, for her time, an amazing amount of support from professionals, patients and concerned citizens, but for the most part the public at large was indifferent.

Not so today. The public is waking up. People all over the planet are questioning authority as never before. We see political systems, once thought totally impervious to change, vanishing overnight. Eastern Europe is free. The Berlin wall has fallen. The Soviet Union no longer exists. For the first time there is a real possibility of peace in the Middle East.

The way we view ourselves, our relationship to our environment, our institutions – in short, the nature of reality – is in the process of redefinition. As we enter a new millennium, old belief systems are dying. Some call it a paradigm shift, a new order. One thing is certain; the stakes are tremendous.

Will the defenders of the old prevail? Will the FDA be successful in limiting your access to alternative therapies? If recent events point to the eventual outcome of dated bureaucracies then we would have to say no. It is more than likely that what you are witnessing with this latest assault by the FDA is the dying gasp of an obsolete institution desperately trying to survive rather than serve.

Already tens of thousands of people around the country have mobilized in an attempt to block the new FDA regulations. Their voices have been heard. Presently, a bill has been proposed in the United States Senate called the Dietary Supplement, Health and Education Act of 1993.

(S. 784. H. R. 1709, Hatch/Richardson.)

The bill in effect will limit the power the FDA has to regulate *herbs* and vitamins, and allow manufacturers or distributors to make truthful health claim for supplements. Its purpose is to preserve your right to have access to dietary supplements and all accurate information about their benefits.

The bill has wide support in both the Senate and the House of Representatives, but it's by no means a done deal. Much of the bill's future depends on what *you* do, right now! Make your feelings known. Write to your senator or congress person and tell them that you want the new bill (S. 784. H.R. 1709, Hatch/Richardson) passed. Find out where they stand!

The Ojibwa believe that history is not linear but circular. Could they be right? The dawn of a new age may be upon us, an age in which the wisdom of our not so distant past will be rediscovered. An age where nature is once again respected and revered, where healing is seen as a total process encompassing the body, mind and spirit. Where mystery and magic are afforded a place in our lives, where we once again understand that we are all part of one "Great Spirit," the source of all things, the indivisible, ultimate reality of the entire universe. You can be part of the vanguard of this new age; you can help usher it in. You need only open your mind to the infinite possibilities of your own life and the "Great Spirit" that sustains it.

Vaya Con Dios.

Section Four

Appendix
Exhibits
Testimonials

EXHIBITS

EXHIBIT ONE:

These three letters are certified copies of correspondence between: Dr. Banting and Rene Caisse, Dr. Banting and Mr. Wilbert Richards, Mayor of Bracebridge, and again, Dr. Banting and Rene Caisse.

Apparently the Mayor had also written to Dr. Banting in support of Rene Caisse.

As was stated in section one, Dr. Banting (the co-discoverer of insulin!) was a highly respected physician. It would be logical to assume that Dr. Banting would not have offered Rene the use of his facilities to test Essiac unless he was absolutely convinced that she was on to something.

COPY

Reply to
   Department of Medical Research
   Banting Institute

UNIVERSITY of TORONTO
Toronto 5, Canada

July 23rd, 1936.

Miss Rene Caisse,
Bracebridge,
Ont.

Dear Miss Caisse,

        I just returned from attending the Canadian
Medical Association meetings in Victoria, B.C. yesterday,
and this afternoon I saw Dr. Faulkner, the Minister of Health,
who has requested that I get in touch with you with regard to
tests being carried out on your treatment for cancer.

        I have told the Honourable Minister of
Health that this laboratory is prepared to do the following:

   (1) Provide you with mice inoculated with mouse
       sarcoma.

   (2) Provide you with chickens inoculated with Rous
       sarcoma.

   (3) These animals will be placed at your disposal in
       the laboratory between the hours of 9 and 5 daily,
       except Sundays and holidays, so that you may treat
       them as you wish.

   (4) You will not be asked to divulge any secret
       concerning your treatment.

   (5) All experimental results must be submitted to me
       for my approval before being announced to anyone,
       including the newspapers, or published in medical
       journals.

   (6) If necessary, special arrangements will be made
       for the special treatment of the animals during
       Sundays and week-ends.

        If You desire that the tests be made under these
conditions, I would be glad to hear from you at your earliest
convenience, so that arrangements can be made.

        With regard to the fifth clause, I wish you to
understand that this is the working arrangement we have with
all other members of the Department; since I have to take the
responsibility of the laboratory, I have to know what is being
reported.

                                    F. G. Banting

                        Yours very truly,

UNIVERSITY OF TORONTO

TORONTO 5, CANADA

August 4th, 1936.

Mr. Wilbert Richards,
Bracebridge,
Ont.

My dear Mayor Richards,

      Your letter of July 25th, concerning Miss Rene Caisse, is received.

      I saw Miss Caisse on Monday, July 27th, and had a talk with her concerning the carrying on of work at Bracebridge. No doubt she has told you the result of this conversation.

      In my opinion it would be impossible for you to adequately test Miss Caisse's cancer treatment in Bracebridge. As I explained to Miss Caisse, I would personally not take any responsibility for work done outside of the laboratory.

      The whole matter was previously discussed with the Honourable Dr. Faulkner, and we are still prepared to test Miss Caisse's treatment under the arrangements set forth in my letter to her.

Yours very truly,

F. G. Banting

F.G. BANTING, M.D.

FGB.M.

COPY

Reply to
  Department of Medical Research
    Banting Institute

                    UNIVERISTY of TORONTO
                    TORONTO 5, Canada

                                        August 11th, 1936.

Miss Rene M. Caisse,
Bracebridge,
Ontario.

Dear Miss Caisse,

            Your letter of August 5th. is
received.

            I think you will regret that you
have not availed yourself of the offer made by this
laboratory to test your treatment for cancer.
However, you must make the decision, and if at
some future time you again decide to have the
treatment investigated, I am sure that Doctor
Faulkner and myself would re-consider the matter.

                        Yours very truly F. G. Banting

FGB.M.
                            F.G. Banting, M.D.

EXHIBIT TWO:

The 1981 Post-Gazette Humanitarian Award. Please read it. You'll get a vivid picture of Rene's partner, Dr. Charles A. Brusch, the remarkable man who helped perfect the old Indian herbal formula and believed so strongly in its power to "cure" cancer.

The Post Gazette is one of Boston's leading newspapers.

1981 Post-Gazette Humanitarian Award

Dr. Charles Armao Brusch

REPRINT

By Lillian Bono

Hippocrates, a Greek philosopher who lived 400 B.C. is said to be the father of medicine. He is the man who gave the world the famous oath that all doctors of medicine take as they rise above other mortals and become the healers of men.

Although these people of great learning are supervised by government agencies, they have a larger and more important agency within themselves that guides them in their pursuits, one that is all encompassing, one that is all forgiving. A doctor has to be everything to everyone and in order to maintain high ideals, a medical person needs to work harder each day.

Such is the make-up of Charles Armao Brusch, a brilliant man who has done much to create a better life for many. Not only is he a person able to recognize and diagnose ailments but he believes in preventative medicine. While his ideals are futuristic, they are filled with love of mankind and dedication to many causes.

Born to Anthony and Mary (Boscia) Brusch of Troy, New York, he is true to his Sicilian heritage. Brusch is the sort of person who will not leave any stone unturned in order to achieve a project and is always engaged in some form of research to benefit others. Educated in the Troy Public School system, he is a graduate of St. Lawrence University, Class of 1934 with a Bachelor of Science. He obtained his medical degree from Tufts University Medical School.

His pursuits were not always mental ones. In his youth he was well known as an expert athlete. While in high school, his extra curricular activities included basketball, track, football and tennis, while in college he excelled in football and wrestling. He was an intern at Mercy Hospital in Springfield, Massachusetts, a famous city -- famous because several well known Italo-Americans came from that part of the state including a former governor of the Bay State.

He established his practice of general medicine in Cambridge, Massachusetts and by 1950 founded the Brusch Medical Center in that city with his brother, the late Dr. Joseph Brusch. As Medical Director of the Center, he attracted the attention of many people all over the country, when he set up the first clinic in Massachusetts to conduct acupuncture research.

He's a writer also and published numerous articles, presenting these papers before groups of peers and at seminars throughout the world. Some include an introduction to the History of Chemistry (American Journal of Pharmacology, November 1955), Combined Treatment of Gastroduodenal Ulcers (Review of Gastoenterology, 1940) and many articles dealing with arthritis, nutrition and allergies.

He is listed with the Community Leaders of America, National Encyclopedia of America (biography), International Biography, Blue Book, National Social Directory, Who's Who in the East, Who's Who in North America, Wisdom Society, Italian

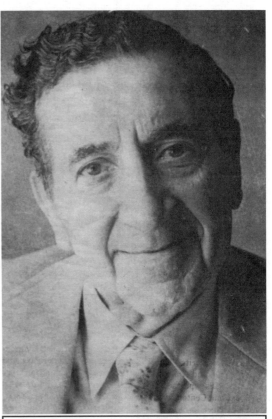

Dr. Charles Armao Brusch, our 1981 Humanitarian Award Recipient. He is a gifted man who has done much to improve the lot of his fellowmmen.

Literary Society, Who's Who of Italian Origin in America, Who's Who of Italian Origin in Massachusetts, The American Catholic Biography, Academia Tiberia Scientific and Historical Society (Rome), Citizens Rights Association of Massachusetts, Guest Biography: Out standing Citizens of North America, Recipient of Stella della Solidarieta Italiana (Star of Solidarity), Order of Knighthood from the Italian Government: Commander, Military and Hospital Order of St. Lazarus of Jerusalem; Knight of Malta; Knight of the Order of Don Orione; and Supreme Commander of the Order of St. George.

He is a member of the American Medical Association, Massachusetts Medical Society, Cambridge Medical

Continued on A - 2

Improvement Society, Massachusetts Federation of Physicians, American Association of Clinical Counselors, American Industrial Association, American Geriatric Society, Internal Protologic Society, Society of Physical Medicine, Mass. Public Health Society, American Assn. of Physicians and Surgeons, American Medical Writers Assn., Royal Academy of Medicine, Boston Tufts Club, St. Lawrence Gridiron Club, Huxley Institute, and is a director of Hearing Dog Foundation as well as a member of many other societies and associations.

As a physician, he is on the staff of the Cambridge Hospital, Santa Maria Hospital, Central Hospital and Longwood Hospital, all located in the Boston/Cambridge area of Massachusetts. Although he has little time for socializing, Dr. Brusch belongs to the Longwood Cricket and Tennis Club, Shady Hill Tennis Club and Nashua Country Club.

In selecting Dr. Brusch as its 1981 "Humanitarian Award" recipient, the Post-Gazette Board of Directors knew that this was a man of honor and integrity had a background that could speak for itself. Brusch is a person who has come a long way. He has worked very hard to achieve the success he enjoys today. He has received many special citations for outstanding work. The City Council of Cambridge recognized him for outstanding service to the sick of the city and students of the schools. The Governor's Council commended him for thirty plus years of unexcelled medicare care to the citizens of the Common wealth of Massachusetts and for professional achievement and philanthropic works of exceptional caliber.

He was knighted by Pope Paul VI and the University of Mayaguez, Puerto Rico cited him for outstanding work in medicine and surgery as well as leadership in scientific medical research. The Dante Alighieri Society has recognized him for his literary, philanthropic and medical contributions. He has been equally cited by the Shamrock Charitable Club, Order of Lazarus,/Order of St. George.

He has served on the Israel Histradut Awards Dinner Committee several times and was quoted in "Get Well Naturally" by Linda Clark. Dr. Robert C. Atkins gave him an honorable mention in "Doctor Atkins Nutrition Breakthrough."

He is an Honorary Director of the Orphans of Italy, Director, North Cambridge Cooperative Bank, former Chairman, current Director Don Orione Home, (E. Boston). Honorary Director of the noted Muscular Dystrophy Assn., former Regional Director, Tufts Medical Alumni Drive, Former Trustee, Brighton Five Cents Savings Bank, Chairman, Board of Trustees, Public Health Welfare Hospital, Honorary Chairman, Boys' Town of Italy, Former Program Chairman, Tufts Medical School, 1934, Honorary Man-of-the-Year, former V.P. of Dante Alighieri Society, Honorary Member, Irish Talent Club, and Honorary Man-of-the-Year, Shamrock Charitable Society.

Dr. and Mrs. Charles A. Brusch. The lovely and very talented Mrs. Brusch is the former Glendora Jane MacKenzie and an artist in her own right.

He built the Infant of Prague Chapel in Brookline New Hampshire, founded the first prepaid medical plan, Electrical union #103, 1955 in Cambridge, distributed the first commercial injection of the polio vaccine in the United States and is the founder of the first medical clinic for the Order of St. George in the Western Hemisphere.

Dr. Brusch is a man of many talents and his home life has been very happy too. He was married to the late Dr. Margaret Lynch Brusch, head of the History Department of Cambridge High and Latin. Dr. Margaret Lynch Brusch was a well known personality whose background was almost as glorious as her husband's. She was deceased in 1966. Recently, Dr. Brusch has remarried. His present wife, Glendora Jane MacKenzie is as lovely as she is beautiful.

He has a son Dr. John L. Brusch and a daughter May Elizabeth Brusch Mulkeen.

Dr. Brusch personifies what America is all about. His success is due to hard work -- his recognition is a direct result of dedication to mankind and love of family is something that he was born with. The warmth he projects is real and many have benefited through his intelligent approach to the many ills that hinder us all from time to time.

To meet Dr. Brusch is an experience -- it was for me and my impression was that he is a rare person, the type that comes about once in a lifetime.

The oath he uttered a half a century ago has created a giant, the sort that history books are made of. Dr. Brusch, is certainly a humanitarian per se.

EXHIBIT THREE:

This document written in 1982 by Dr. Charles A. Brusch is a summation of his research and work with Essiac. It's rather convincing testimony from one of America's most esteemed physicians that Essiac does in fact "cure" cancer. The last paragraph says it all:

"The results we obtained with thousands of patients of various races, sexes and ages, will all types of cancer definitely proves Essiac to be a cure for cancer. Studies done in four laboratories in the United States and one or more in Canada also fortify this claim."

Dr. Brusch does not mince words.

BRUSCH MEDICAL ASSOCIATES INC.

843 MASSACHUSETTS AVENUE

CAMBRIDGE. MASSACHUSETTS 02139

TEL. (617) 864-1640

July 30/8 *R-5:*

RESEARCH ON ESSIAC

Charles A. Brusch, M.D.

Essiac is an herb formula made from several different herbs with no additives. It was first.introduced about seventy years ago by Rene Caisse, a nurse in Bracebridge, Ontario, Canada.

This Essiac formula was used for the treatment of cancer and was also researched by numerous doctors who treated thousands of patients. These treatments have been documented by doctors, by individuals who have been cured, and by members of patients' families who can testify to the effects of Essiac. Documentation included many cases, including a history of the physical examination, laboratory findings, x-rays, clinical findings and progress notes.

In 1958 Rene Caisse began working at the Brusch Medical Research Center. At that time we commenced our research project to prove the merits of Essiac in the treatment of cancer. We used the herbal medicine as an oral treatment: two ounces of Essiac each night in one-half to one glass of warm water, with no other medication, on an empty stomach. A little later we.were anxious to find.out what the active ingredients were. So we experimented with injectible solutions, each vial containing a different herb in the Essiac formula. We failed to isolate a single outstanding herb. We found out that reactions and results were not so good so we stopped injections with the isolated herbs and returned to using the oral medication. Experimenting with the single herbal injections proved to us that best results were obtained by the combination of herbs contained in Essiac and not in one single active herb.

Good results obtained by taking the Essiac herbal medicine included cessation of pain, increased appetite, weight gain, feeling of well being which reflected improved emotional attitudes.regarding depression, anxiety, and fear, and prolongation of life. Results improved with the continuance of the Essiac medication.

The Essiac Research Program at Brusch Medical Center was carried on by Rene Caisse and myself; Director of Research; by Dr. Charles Mc Clure, former Professor of Gastroenterology and Research at Boston University Medical School and Peter B. Brigham Hospital, a member of Who's Who in World Medicine; by Dr. P. Pappas, former Professor of Urology at Tufts Medical School, affiliated with New England Medical Center; by Dr. George Ceresia, PH. D., Professor of Chemistry, Albany School of Chemistry, affiliated with Union University, Schenectedy, New York.

Here at Brusch Medical Research Center, animal experimentation was conducted with good results on 35 mice. We decided to have experimentation with animals rechecked so additional experimentation was conducted at the Sloan-Kettering Institute of Cancer in New York and by

Bioran Blood Chemistry Laboratory in Cambridge, Massachusetts.

With each patient who was a candidate for Essiac treatment we conducted a thorough physical examination, including blood analysis, EKG, x-rays, and any other clinical test that seemed pertinent.

Whenever a patient was referred to us we always obtained a history of past treatments and when possible, we would send to the doctor concerned a history of results obtained at Brusch Medical Center. Oftentimes, when the patient returned to his home town or state, the attending doctor would send us progress notes.

The Sloan-Kettering studies with mice were done in June, 1975. One hundred eighty mice were used in the study that showed a recession of growth of tumors.

We were satisfied with these results although we know that results obtained in animals do not always equate response in humans. In the case of animals, tumors are bred in selected species and so animal tumors are definitely different from tumors in humans. In humans we deal with many complicated issues; often other diseases such as arthritis, allergies, diabetes, nervous tension are present and affect the tumorous condition, something that was not present in selected animals.

In summary, Essiac, a non-toxic herbal formula used in the treatment of cancer is not incompatible for use with other medications, radiation, chemotherapy, x-rays, or any other known treatment. It can be used for an indefinite period of time, does not spoil, is easy to administer, is inexpensive, can be administerd by a doctor or taken by prescription.

At one period of experimentation we also used a double blind study in which we used other herb formulas, all of which proved to be inferior to Essiac. In some cases we used medication in form of tablets or placebos with no results.

I feel that the experimentation with Essiac was an outstanding piece of work considering the wonderful effects achieved by using Essiac. For over 65 years the formula was used constantly by doctors, proving its merits of healing and non-toxic effects. Studies carried on in Canada and in the United States, two different countries, gave the same results.

In a June, 1982 medical radio program known as PRN, fakery in research was aired, showing that research projects on cancer, some done independently and some by medical schools, gave many false statistics in projects for which millions of dollars had been appropriated. We had

no grants given to us; all studies, including those done in two different countries, in different laboratories, by different doctors, were conducted with strictly ethical procedures and everything could be re-checked.

The results we obtained with thousands of patients of various races, sexes, and ages, with all types of cancer, definitely prove Essiac to be a cure for cancer. All studies done in four laboratories in the United States and one or more in Canada fortify this claim.

Charles A. Brusch, M.D.

EXHIBIT FOUR:

As a physician, it's one thing to say Essiac is a cure for cancer because you've seen it heal other people. It quite another to believe so strongly in its powers that when the dreaded disease finds its way into your own body, you are then willing to abandon all other known therapies in favor of Essiac!

This notarized document speaks for itself.

CHARLES A. BRUSCH, M.D.
15 GROZIER RD.
CAMBRIDGE, MASSACHUSETTS 02138

April 6, 1990

TO WHOM IT MAY CONCERN:

Many years have gone by since I first experienced the use of ESSIAC with my patients who were suffering from many varied forms of Cancer.

I personally monitored the use of this old therapy along with Rene Caisse R.N. whose many successes were widely reported. Rene worked with me at my medical clinic in Cambridge, Massachusetts and where, under the supervision of 18 of my many medical doctors on staff, she proceeded with a series of treatments on terminal Cancer patients and laboratory mice and together we refined and perfected her formula.

On mice it has been shown to cause a decided recession of the mass and a definite change in cell formation.

Clinically, on patients suffering from pathologically proven Cancer, it reduces pain and causes a recession in the growth. Patients gained weight and showed a great improvement in their general health. Their elimination improved considerably and their appetite became whetted.

Remarkably beneficial results were obtained even on those cases at the "end of the road" where it proved to prolong life and the "quality" of that life.

In some cases, if the tumor didn't disappear, it could be surgically removed after ESSIAC with less risk of mestastases resulting in new outbreaks.

Hemorrhage has been rapidly brought under control in many difficult cases, open lesions of lip and breast responded to treatment, and patients with Cancer of the stomach have returned to normal activity among many other remembered cases. Also, intestinal burns from radiation were healed and damage replaced, and it was found to greatly improve whatever the condition.

All these patient cases were diagnosed by reputable physicians and surgeons.

I do know that I have witnessed in my clinic and know of many other cases where ESSIAC was the therapy used, a treatment which brings about restoration through destroying the tumor tissue and improving the mental outlook which re-establishes physiological function.

_____

I endorse this therapy even today for I have in fact cured my own Cancer, the original site of which was the lower bowel, through ESSIAC alone.

My last complete examination, where I was examined throughout the intestinal tract while hospitalized (August, 1989) for a hernia problem, no sign of malignancy was found.

Medical documents validate this.

I have taken ESSIAC every day since my diagnosis (1984) and my recent examination has given me a clear bill of health.

I remained a partner with Rene Caisse until her death in 1978 and was the only person who had her complete trust and to whom she confided her knowledge and "know-how" of what she named "ESSIAC."

Others have imitated, but a minor success rate should never be accepted when the true therapy is available.

Executed as a legal document.

_____
            Charles A. Brusch, M.D.

Signed, Sealed and Delivered
in the Presence of

Witness:

_____
Address: 2360 Massachusetts Avenue
         Cambridge, MA 02140
Occupation: Banker
_____

Date: April 11, 1990
_____

_____
                          Notary

My Commission expires:_____

                    William E. Moriarty
                       Notary Public
            My Commission Expires Oct. 5, 1990

EXHIBIT FIVE:

This exhibit consists of two documents. The first document, which begins: To whom it may concern--
is a memorialization of the *understood* partnership between Dr. Brusch and Rene Caisse. It was drawn up at Rene's insistence and duly signed six days before her October 26, 1976, meeting was David Fingard.

The second document is the agreement between Resperin and Rene Caisse, signed on October 26, 1976.

The agreement is somewhat lengthy, but is worth the trouble of reading. There is much talk of the "sealed" envelope which contained the "formula!" If contracts can be dramatic this one has its moments:

"Rene M. Caisse also agrees that upon the signing of this agreement Mr. Fingard (but only Mr. Fingard) shall have the right to open the said sealed envelope containing the particulars of the Essiac treatment and the formula for and ingredients of all medication comprised therein."

But, alas, as you may already know, it was *much ado about nothing.*

                                        293 Hiram Street
                                        Bracebridge
                                        Ontario, Canada

To Whom It May Concern:

     I, Rene Caisse, agree to give to Doctor Charles A. Brusch,

831 Massachusetts AVenue, Cambridge, Massachusetts 02139, 1% share

when the Essiac formula is marketed.

     In case of my death before that time, Doctor Charles Brusch

is to receive 2% share.

     In case the formula is not developed, it is to be returned to

Doctor Charles Brusch, Cambridge, Massachusetts 02139, in order that

in my name he may continue research with Essiac in the Rene Caisse

Cancer Foundation.

     This arrangement is made in appreciation of the work that Doctor

Charles A. Brusch has done as my co-worker.

                     Signature   _Rene M Caisse_____

                     Date   ___10/20/1977_____

AGREEMENT made as of the 26th day of October, 1977.

BETWEEN:

RESPERIN CORPORATION LIMITED,
a company incorporated under the laws
of the Province of Ontario

(hereinafter called "Resperin")

OF THE FIRST PART

- and -

DAVID FINGARD, of the Municipality
of Metropolitan Toronto, in the Province
of Ontario

(hereinafter called "Mr. Fingard")

OF THE SECOND PART

- and -

RENE M. CAISSE, of the Town of
Bracebridge, in the Province of Ontario,
Registered Nurse

(hereinafter called Rene M. Caisse)

OF THE THIRD PART

WHEREAS Rene M. Caisse represents and warrants to

Resperin and Mr. Fingard that she has developed and has sole and

exclusive proprietary rights to a treatment for the alleviation and cure

of cancer (such treatment being hereinafter referred to as the "Essiac"

treatment);

AND WHEREAS Rene M. Caisse also represents and

warrants to Resperin and Mr. Fingard that she has not disclosed to

any other person or company any particulars of the Essiac treatment

the formula for or ingredients of any medication comprised therein;

AND WHEREAS Rene M. Caisse represents and warrants to Resperin and Mr. Fingard that a sealed envelope containing all particulars of the Essiac treatment and the formula for and ingredients of all medication comprised therein has been lodged in trust with the Lieutenant Governor of the Province of Ontario under a trust agreement (hereinafter called the "Trust Agreement") and that such Trust Agreement provides, inter alia, that Rene M. Caisse may terminate the said Trust Agreement and recover the said sealed envelope containing all particulars of the Essiac treatment and the formula for and ingredients of all medication comprised therein at any time;

AND WHEREAS Rene M. Caisse and Resperin have agreed to co-operate in the promotion of the Essiac treatment for use throughout the world in the alleviation and cure of cancer all on and subject to the terms of this agreement;

NOW THEREFORE THIS AGREEMENT WITNESSETH THAT in consideration of the premises and of the mutual covenants herein contained and of the sum of One Dollar ($1.00) of lawful money of Canada now paid to each of the parties hereto by the other (the receipt of which is hereby acknowledged) the parties covenant and agree as follows:

1. Rene M. Caisse hereby agrees to forthwith terminate the Trust Agreement and to deliver the sealed envelope containing all particulars of the Essiac treatment and the formula for and ingredients

dication comprised therein to Mr. Fingard, on behalf of Resperin, Rene M. Caisse hereby sells, assigns, transfers and sets over unto Resperin all her right, title and interest in and to the Essiac treatment and the formula for and ingredients of all medication comprised therein, subject to the terms and conditions hereinafter set forth.

2.   Rene M. Caisse also agrees that upon the signing of this agreement Mr. Fingard (but only Mr. Fingard) shall have the right to open the said sealed envelope containing the particulars of the Essiac treatment and the formula for and ingredients of all medication comprised therein. Mr. Fingard agrees, however, that upon receipt of the said sealed envelope from Rene M. Caisse he will immediately lodge the same and maintain the same in safekeeping in trust with Mr. Stephen B. Roman or Mr. Edgar A. Eaton and that the terms of such trust shall be to the effect that, during the six month period referred to in paragraph 4 hereof, the trustee will grant access to the said sealed envelope only to Mr. Fingard (or in the event of the death of Mr. Fingard during the said six month period, then to one of the persons mentioned in paragraph 5 hereof) and that such trust shall not be terminable during the said six month period but may be terminated at any time after the expiration of the said six month period by Mr. Fingard or by Resperin or by one of the persons mention in paragraph 5. hereof.

3.   Notwithstanding the provisions of paragraph 1 hereof, each of Resperin and Mr. Fingard hereby covenants and agrees that it and he will not communicate any particulars of the Essiac treatment or the

...la for or ingredients of any medication comprised therein to any

...rson, whether or not an officer, director or shareholder of Resperin

unless and until Resperin shall not have given to Rene M. Caisse a

notice in writing referred to in paragraph 7 hereof. In the event

Resperin does not give such notice in writing to Rene M. Caisse,

Resperin and Mr. Fingard shall no longer be under any obligation of

non-disclosure under this paragraph 2.

4.   Resperin hereby agrees that during the period of not more

than six months after the date hereof (hereinafter called the "six months'

period") it will conduct a medical re-evaluation of the Essiac treatment

using such test methods as it deems appropriate in its sole discretion

and Rene M. Caissé hereby agrees to co-operate fully with Resperin

in the conduct of such re-evaluation and to provide Resperin with all

information at her disposal with respect to patients who have been

given the Essiac treatment. Such re-evaluation shall be carried on

by Resperin in such places as it may reasonably decide but if it should

be necessary for Rene M. Caisse to travel from her home to the place of

such re-evaluation, Resperin shall pay all of her reasonable transporta-

tion expenses.

5.   Rene M. Caisse understands and agrees that the medical

re-evaluation of the Essiac treatment herein provided for shall be

conducted on behalf of Resperin by and under the sole auspices of

Mr. Fingard, Dr. Charles Brusch, Dr. E. Thomas French, Dr.

Matthew Dymond and Dr. P. B. Rynard. Rene M. Caisse also agrees

...s advised by Mr. Fingard that, in his view, it has become
...ry for the purposes of such medical re-evaluation of the Essiac
...tment to disclose to one or more of the individuals referred to in
the previous sentence one or more aspects of the Essiac treatment or
the formula for or ingredients of any medication comprised therein,
she will not unreasonably withhold her written consent to the furnishing
of such information to such person upon the request of Mr. Fingard.

6.   During the six months' period Resperin shall pay to Rene
M. Caisse a fee of $250 per week in addition to any expenses paid to
her under paragraph 4 hereof.

7.   If at the end of the six months period, Resperin is not
satisfied in its sole discretion with the results of the medical re-evaluation
of the Essiac treatment referred to in paragraph 4 hereof, Resperin shall
give a notice in writing to Rene M. Caisse advising her of such fact, and
shall at that time execute and deliver to Rene M. Caisse an unconditional
transfer and assignment of all the right, title and interest of Resperin in
and to the Essiac treatment and the formula for and ingredients of all
medication comprised therein and Mr. Fingard shall arrange on behalf
of Resperin to return to Rene M. Caisse the envelope containing particulars
of the Essiac treatment and the formula for and ingredients of any
medication comprised therein together with a complete report on the
re-evaluation including all case histories.

8.   If at the end of the six months' period Resperin has not
given to Rene M. Caisse the notice in writing referred to in paragraph 7

of it shall be deemed to have been satisfied with the results of its medical re-evaluation of the Essiac treatment referred to in paragraph 4 hereof. In such event, Resperin and Rene M. Caisse agree that they will co-operate fully in the promotion of the Essiac treatment for use throughout the world in the alleviation and cure of cancer and that from and after the expiration of the six months' period Resperin shall pay to Rene M. Caisse, as and by way of a continuing royalty payment, an amount equal to 2% of the gross revenue received by Resperin arising out of the said promotion of the Essiac treatment.

9. In the event of the death of Mr. Fingard during the six months' period Rene M. Caisse agrees that the trustee referred to in paragraph 2 hereof may communicate all particulars of the Essiac treatment and the formula for and the ingredients of all medication comprised therein to any one (but not more than one without the consent of Rene M. Caisse) of the persons mentioned in paragraph 4 hereof.

10. In the event of the communication of any particulars of the Essiac treatment or the formula for and ingredients of the medication comprised therein to any person other than Mr. Fingard as hereby permitted during the six month's period, Resperin shall cause to be executed and delivered to Rene M. Caisse an agreement signed by such person in which he agrees to be bound by the terms of this agreement.

11. This agreement shall enure to the benefit of and be binding upon the parties hereto and their respective heirs, executors, administrators, successors and assigns. However, Resperin shall

e entitled to assign its interest in this agreement during the afore-
aid six months' period to any other person, firm or corporation without
the express written consent of Rene M. Caisse.

12.   In the event that any party to this agreement fails for any
reason to fulfill and discharge such party's responsbilities under this
agreement or fails to adhere to the terms and conditions set out herein,
the other party or parties shall be entitled to take all appropriate legal
recourse against the defaulting party.

           IN WITNESS WHEREOF the parties hereto have executed
this agreement.

                                        RESPERIN CORPORATION LIMITED

                                        By _____

                                                                    C.S.
                                        _____

SIGNED, SEALED AND DELIVERED)
)
in the presence of   )
) _____
)   David Fingard
)
)
)
) _____
)   Rene M. Caisse

EXHIBIT SIX:

This letter to Dr. M.B. Dymond, President of Resperin, from Dr. Ian W.D. Henderson, Director, Bureau of Drugs, spells out the requirements for the pre-clinical submission for Essiac.

The letter also speaks of the "investigators who are qualified to use the drug." (the doctors who would be conducting the clinical testing.) It specifically refers to Form HPB 3082 and HPB 3005 "which should be completed by each qualified investigator and returned to the Resperin Corporation Ltd."

Unfortunately we have not been given access to these two forms but understand through reliable sources that the requirements to be adhered to by the "investigating" doctors were extremely rigid and time consuming, far more than most doctors were willing to put up with over an extended period of time.

Tower "B",
355 River Road,
VANIER, Ontario.
K1A 1B8

June 22, 1978

R·6

M.B. Dymond, M.D.,   } RESPERIN
Drawer 89,
PORT PERRY, Ontario.
L0B 1N0

Dear Dr. Dymond:

        Receipt is acknowledged of your letter of June 17,
1978, requesting information about the requirements of the
Food and Drug Regulations which must be met before Essiac
can be rleeased for clinical testing in Canada.

        The preclinical submission for Essiac should consist
of two copies of completed Form HPB 3802 accompanied by the
following additional data required by Section C.08.005 (1)
(a) of the Regulations:

"(v)   the results of investigations made to support the
            clinical use for the new drug,

 (vi)   the contra-indications and precautions known in
            respect of the new drug and the suggested treatment
            of overdosage of the new drug,

 (vii)   the methods, equipment, plant and controls used in
            the manufacture, processing and packaging of the
            new drug,

 (viii)   the tests applied to control the potency, purity
            and safety of the new drug and

 (ix)   the name and qualifications of all investigators
            to whom the drug is to be sold and the names of all
            institutions in which the investigations are to be
            carried out."

        The labels used for Essiac should carry the statements
"Investigational Drug" and "To Be Used by Qualified Investigators Only."

R·7

Dr. M.B. Dymond   June 22, 1978

     The Regulations also state that Essiac may be distributed
only to investigators who are qualified to use the drug, for
the sole purpose of clinical testing, to obtain evidence with
respect to the safety, dosage and effectiveness of the drug.

     You will find enclosed several copies of Form HPB 3082
and HPB 3005. The latter (Statement of Investigator of New
Drugs) should be completed by each qualified investigator and
returned to the Respirin Corporation Ltd.

     I assure you and the Board again that all information
in the preclinical submission for Essiac will be kept in
strict confidence by the members of my staff who are qualified
to review and evaluate such data. The file will be marked
"CONFIDENTIAL".

     I am looking forward to receiving your preclinical
submission for Essiac in the very near future.

                Yours sincerely,

                signed.

                Ian W.D. Henderson, M.D.,
                Director,
                Bureau of Drugs.

Encls.

NRS/tm

EXHIBIT SEVEN:

This *internal memorandum* (April 9, 1981) of the Health Protection Branch is extremely instructive concerning their hidden agenda towards Essiac. It clearly states *why* The Health Protection Branch felt Resperin's clinical testing was inadequate, and *why* that inadequacy would make it *impossible* to determine if Essiac was in fact effective against cancer. It leaves no doubt about the real reasons behind the Health Protection Branch's ultimate decision to shut down Resperin's clinical testing program. *Reasons that were never articulated to the public.*

This exhibit, as with many of the exhibits herein, was obtained visavis the Freedom of Information Act.

BRIEFING INFORMATION ON ESSIAC

H.52

Essiac, a herbal product, intended for treatment of cancer and produced by the Resperin Corporation, was conditionally cleared for clinical trials in 1978. At that time, the Health Protection Branch took no objection to the distribution of Essiac to qualified investigators for the purpose of clinical testing to obtain evidence with respect to its safety, dosage and effectiveness. This decision was based on the understanding that Essiac will be manufactured under appropriate controls as required by the Food and Drug Regulations and that the clinical trials with Essiac will be monitored by a national agency concerned with the therapy of cancer, in order to arrive at scientifically valid data to substantiate the effectiveness of this drug in treatment of malignant disease(s).

In spite of repeated reminders from the Health Protection Branch, the drug manufacturer failed to implement the above conditions. Essiac was distributed by the Resperin Corporation to some 160 physicians throughout Canada for treatment of cancer patients.

To date, the Health Protection Branch has received a small number of incomplete clinical case reports, but no data which would establish that the product distributed is uniform in composition from batch to batch. Without this information, the results of the clinical studies are impossible to evaluate. Concerns about the clinical use of Essiac and the patient diversion from proven conventional methods of therapy have been repeatedly expressed by members of the medical profession.

H.5

The data presently available on Essiac were recently reviewed independantly by two nongovernment consultants, known medical specialists on cancer treatment. Both consultants found the clinical studies poorly conceived and executed, yielding uninterpretable results. Termination of the clinical trials as currently constituted was recommended by both consultants.

In view of this, the Health Protection Branch on behalf of the Minister, pursuant to Section C.08.005(3) intends to notify the Resperin Corporation that in the interest of public health, the clearance of the investigational new drug submission for Essiac will be cancelled.

It can be expected that this decision will give rise to some accusations that the medical establishment is not prepared to give the drug manufacturer a proper opportunity to establish its therapeutic value. There may also be a negative reaction from cancer victims who are presently taking Essiac and will have their supply cut off. Conversely, the decision will still criticism from the medical profession that the Branch is allowing an unproven drug to be distributed under inappropriate conditions.

Health Protection Branch

April 9. 1981 -- 11:15 a.m.

EXHIBIT EIGHT:

The End! Direct from the Minister of Health, Monique Begin, to Dr. M.B. Dymond, President of Resperin Corporation, former *Minister of Health.*

Resperin had blown the opportunity of a lifetime and had at the same time given the Department of Health and Welfare the means by which they could now *finally* put an end to the *Essiac problem,* or so they thought.

The public of course was unaware of what was happening.

CANADA

MINISTER OF NATIONAL HEALTH AND WELFARE

MINISTRE DE LA
SANTE NATIONALE ET DU BIEN-ETRE SOCIAL

OTTAWA, K1A 0K9

AUG
AOU 30 1982

Dr. M.B. Dymond,
President,
Resperin Corporation Limited,
280 Cochrane Street,
Drawer 89,
PORT PERRY, Ontario.
L0B 1N0

Dear Dr. Dymond:

I am writing in regard to your preclinical new drug submission for ESSIAC, IND No. HP-7825. In his letter to you of October 12, 1978, Dr. A.B. Morrison informed you that the Health Protection Branch would take no objection to the distribution of ESSIAC to qualified investigators provided certain conditions were met. These conditions included the following:

1. attempts would be made to isolate and identify the active antineoplastic substance or substances in ESSIAC,

2. the antineoplastic activity of ESSIAC or its components would be investigated and adequately established in suitable biological systems or organisms,

3. the clinical trials would be monitored by a national agency concerned with therapy of cancer in order to arrive at scientifically valid data to substantiate the effectiveness of this drug in the treatment of malignant disease,

... 2

R. 69

Dr. M.B. Dymond

4. a description of the quality control
procedures used to ensure lot to lot
uniformity of the raw materials would
b⁻ provided, and

5. the results of stability studies would
be provided.

Despite repeated requests, these conditions have ✗
not been fulfilled.

In addition, you have failed to comply with the ✗
requirements of paragraph C.08.005(1)(c) of the Food
and Drug Regulations.

I am therefore notifying you, pursuant to subsection
C.08.005(3) of the Regulations, that in my opinion it is ✶
in the interest of public health to prohibit further sales
✶ of ESSIAC. Thus any further sales of ESSIAC would be a
violation of subsection C.08.005(4) of the Regulations.

Please note that the Food and Drugs Act defines
"sell" to include "distribute". ✗

Should you decide to make arrangements to fulfill
the above conditions and file another submission with
the Health Protection Branch, the matter of further sales
of ESSIAC would of course be considered.

Yours truly,

Original Signed by
Copie originale signée par

Monique Bégin

EXHIBIT NINE:

This letter from the Health Protection Branch to Dr. A.V. Neufeld should give you some idea why many doctors, at first enthusiastic about Essiac's real possibilities, would be reluctant to try to obtain it under the Emergency Drug Release Act.

Not only are the requirements for obtaining Essiac rather extensive, especially to a doctor who has a hard time with paper work, as most do, the Health Protection Branch goes on to inform the prospective doctor that Essiac does not work. Why it does not work is based on the Health Protection Branch's total misrepresentation of the facts!

Health and Welfare
Canada

Santé et Bien-être social
Canada

Health Protection
Branch

Direction générale de la
protection de la santé

Place Vanier,
Tower "B",
355 River Road,
Vanier, Ontario.
K1A 1B8

December 31, 1985.

OTTAWA

Dr. A. V. Neufeld,
Dewdney Medical Group,
Suite B,
22195 Dewdney Trk. Rd.,
MAPLE RIDGE, B.C.
V2X 3H7

Dear Doctor Neufeld:

Thank you for your letter dated December 18, 1985 regarding Essiac.

It is stipulated within the Section C.08.010 and C.08.011 of the Food and Drug Regulations that physicians requesting non-marketed drugs must supply the following information to the Health Protection Branch prior to any further shipments. These requirements are as follows:

1. The full medical history including details of prior treatment and full data on the type of malignancy for which Essiac is required.

2. The name and address of the institution or the home address in which Essiac is to be used.

3. Data in your possession with respect to the safety and efficacy of Essiac in clinical trials, all instructions regarding optimal use and knowledge of the ingredients within this herbal product.

It is encumbent upon the Health Protection Branch to inform you of the following facts: Essiac is an infusion [DECOCTION] of the following herbs: Indian Rhubarb, Sheephead Sorrel, Slippery Elm and Burdock. (Turkish Rhubarb) and Watercress etc.

... 2

Given from the Health Protection Branch they have it wrong -

Dr. A. V. Neufeld

In recent usage in Canada about 150 physicians were known to have received supplies for individual patients. The Health Protection Branch contacted these physicians and received replies from 74 concerning 86 patients. The following results were analyzed from these reports: 47 patients reported no benefits; 8 of the reports were not evaluable; 17 patients had died; 1 patient was reported to have had a subjective improvement; 5 patients were reported as requiring less analgesia; 4 patients were said to have an objective response; and 4 patients were in a stable condition. The Health Protection Branch then followed up the 8 patients who according to their physicians had had an objective response or who had remained stable. In early 1982 these patients were re-examined by their physicians and the following results were obtained:

In 3 of the 8 the disease had progressed; 2 had died; and 3 were remaining stable. The 3 stable patients histories were further documented and it is the impression of the Health Protection Branch that in these cases the stability was due to other forms of treatment. The conclusion from these 86 patients must therefore be that Essiac had not altered the progression of cancer in these patients, and did not show any specific benefit with the exception of a possible placebo effect in some cases.

With regard to safety, very few patients have had any symptoms referable to the drug. With occasional batches there was some nausea and vomiting. This was probably due to a variation in composition; to our knowledge this has been corrected.

The distribution of Essiac at this time is authorized on the basis that there is no other appropriate treatment for the patients and that notwithstanding the lack of objective data demonstrating benefit, the treating physician for psychological reasons wishes to have his/her patient use this herbal preparation If you wish to obtain Essiac you can either write my office or call at Area Code 613, Number 993-3231.

Yours sincerely,

J. D. Sproul, M.D.,
Clinical Advisor - Oncology,
Bureau of Human Prescription Drugs.

EXHIBIT TEN:

To suppress the truth is always a risky
and ultimately futile endeavor. No sooner had the Department of Health and
Welfare begun to celebrate the demise of
Essiac then they were to receive this letter from Dr. E. Bruce Hendrick, M.D.

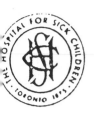
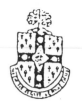

The Hospital for Sick Children
Suite 1502, 555 University Ave.
Toronto, Ontario M5G 1X8
Canada — (416) 597-0808
(416) 598-6425

University of Toronto
Faculty of Medicine
Toronto, Canada

E. Bruce Hendrick, M.D., B.Sc.(MED.), F.R.C.S.(C)
CHIEF OF NEUROSURGERY

PROFESSOR OF SURGERY
DIVISION OF NEUROSURGERY

October 5, 1983

Mme. Monique Begin
Minister of Health & Welfare
House of Commons
Parliament Building
Ottawa, Ontario
K1A 0A1

Dear Mme. Begin:

I am writing this letter in support of a scientific clinical trial of the cancer treatment with the compound known as "Essiac".

At the present time, at the Hospital for Sick Children, there are some 10 patients with surgically treated tumors of the central nervous system, who have escaped from conventional methods of therapy including both radiation and chemotherapy.

The patients who were started on Essiac have at the present time a to limited followup period to reach definite conclusions. However, in 8 of the 10 patients, there has been significant improvement in their neurological state. For further confirmation of the effectiveness of this treatment we'll wait on CAT scans and subsequent investigation.

I am however most impressed with the effectiveness of the treatment and its lack of side effects.

I feel that this method of treatment should be given serious consideration and would benefit from a scientific clinical trial.

Yours sincerely,

E. Bruce Hendrick, M.D., F.R.C.S.(C)
Chief, Division of Neurosurgery

EBH/fm

EXHIBIT ELEVEN:

Elaine Alexander's reasoning was right on target. Besides once again grossly mis-stating the facts about Essiac, this Health Protection Branch Internal Memorandum clearly verifies what she feared:

Any attempt at marketing Essiac as an herbal tea through health food stores would most likely be stopped by the medical authorities because the name Essiac was so closely associated with cancer treatment.

* It is important to note that this document refers to a test conducted at the National Cancer Institute, Bethesda, Maryland, in which Essiac was shown to have no anti tumor activity in mice infected with "mouse sarcoma."

We have been unable to find out the details of this alleged test. But we have included the results of a similar test on Essiac that really did occur, conducted by The Sloan Kettering Institute for Cancer Research, June 10, 1975. (Exhibit 11A). Their findings are certainly different than the supposed findings reported by the Health Protection Branch.

Even though the Sloan Kettering test was flawed in every possible way (See Section One, Page 33.) Essiac was still able to produce some tumor regressions.

BRIEFING INFORMATION ON

ESSIAC AS AN HERBAL TEA

ANTICIPATED QUESTION:

- Why cannot Essiac be sold in Health Food Stores as an herbal tea?

BACKGROUND:

- Essiac is an infusion of tea made from Indian Rhubarb, Sheephead Sorrel, Slippery Elm and Burdock Root.

- In 1978 a Preclinical New Drug Submission was submitted, and despite deficiencies, a Notice of Compliance was granted for Laval University and the Toronto General Hospital to investigate Essiac in cancer patients.

- Subsequently, family practitioners were allowed to supervise treatment with Essiac in patients for whom no other form of treatment was indicated.

- In 1982 these physicians were contacted and reported that in 78 of 87 patients, Essiac showed no benefit. In those where some benefit was claimed, the result could have well been a carryover effect from their prior therapy.

- In 1983 the Health Protection Branch requested the National Cancer Institute (Bethesda, Maryland) to test Essiac in their tumour screening assay system (mouse sarcoma), and their report stated no anti-tumour activity.

CURRENT STATUS:

- No active IND exists currently for Essiac.

- Essiac is being authorized for sale to family practitioners via Emergency Drug authorization.

- Essiac was made until December 1987 by Dr. M. Dymond and his wife, personally, in their home.

- Since December '88 there has been no source of Essiac in Canada.

- A letter from Mr. Stan Darling to Dr. R.C.B. Graham received this week, the response to which has not yet been mailed, notes that

RELEVANT FACTORS:

- Essiac has always been classified as a drug because the Resperin Corporation has made drug claims for this infusion.

- According to the Food and Drugs Act, a substance is a drug when it is a substance or a mixture of substances sold or represented for use in the diagnosis, treatment, investigation or prevention of a disease, disorder, abnormal physical state or the symptoms thereof, etc.

- Essiac has always been represented to be a "cure" for cancer; therefore, it is a drug due to the claim.

SUGGESTED RESPONSE:

- Essiac appears to be entirely non-toxic.

- From the evidence to date Essiac has only a placebo or a psychological effect on cancer patients.

- If Essiac were to be sold in Health Food Stores, the implied claims for this substance could be considered fraudulent, and would also constitute a health hazard with regard to self diagnosis and self treatment of cancer.

Dr. A. Klein (993-1592)
Health Protection Branch
March 17, 1988

LOAN-KETTERING INSTITUTE *for* CANCER RESEARCH

AID S WALKER LABORATORY, 145 BOSTON POST RD., RYE, N.Y 10500   OWENS N Y

June 10, 1975

Mrs. Rene M. Caissee McGaughey
293 Hiram Street
Bracebridge, Ontario
Canada

Dear Mrs. McGaughey:

Enclosed are test data in two experiments indicating some regressions in sarcoma 180 of mice treated with Essiac. With these results we will wish to test enough more that I should ask if you can send more material. If you have questions about the data, please don't hesitate to ask them.

The tests on laetrile did not interfere with the testing of your material.

We are glad to hear you are improving.

Sincerely,

C. Chester Stock, Ph. D.
Vice-President for
Academic Affairs

CCS:mk
encl

EXHIBIT TWELVE:

The 1988, document is a copy of the original partnership agreement between Elaine Alexander and Dr. Charles A. Brusch.

The November 2, 1991 document was presented to the public as means to clarify and reconfirm Dr. Brusch's relationship with Elaine Alexander as the sole and only legal recipient of the "original herbal formula named Essiac."

Apparently a few unscrupulous marketers of so called health products in Canada have tried to dupe the public into believing that they have obtained the "original" Essiac formula authorized by none other than Dr. Charles A. Brusch, himself.

These entirely fallacious claims have caused some confusion in the public mind. This document should, hopefully put an end to both the confusion and the danger attached to purchasing a bogus formula.

CHARLES A. BRUSCH, M.D.
15 GROZIER ROAD
CAMBRIDGE, MASSACHUSETTS 02138

November 2, 1991

TO WHOM IT MAY CONCERN:

This is to verify that through Legal Agreements drawn November 10, 1988 between myself and Canadian broadcaster Elaine E. Alexander of Vancouver, British Columbia; I declare that this above-specified person is the legal recipient of the original Herbal Formula, named "ESSIAC" by the registered nurse Rene Caisse, and with whom I successfully treated patients for many years.

This then confirms the above and also states that I was Rene Caisse's confidant and partner in all matters related to her formulae and the refinement of such through laboratory research in my medical clinic in Cambridge, Massachusetts when Rene Caisse worked with me and we perfected this and related formulae together.

Through this above-mentioned agreement, I confirm that Elaine E. Alexander has in her possession the refined and perfected original formula and the rights to such and, also, the rights to any related formulae of Rene Caisse's and vital "know-how" knowledge and reference documentation connected with such as to proper usage, resulting in the desired optimum results.

I have been approached from many sides to divulge this secret formula and my name has been used in recent broadcasts and publications without my consent, no doubt to authenticate their statements. But I declare unequivocally that this secret formula, and related formulae, was legally given by me to her (as stated above) and only to her.

Executed as a legal document.

Charles A. Brusch, M.D.

CHARLES A. BRUSCH, M.D.
15 GROZIER ROAD
CAMBRIDGE, MASSACHUSETTS 02138

Signed, Sealed and Delivered
in the Presence of Witness:

James F. Culhane

Address: 2360 Mass Ave., Cambridge, MA

Occupation: Bank President

Date: Nov. 4, 1991

Notary

My Commission expires: 10/24/97

WILLIAM E. MORIARTY
NOTARY PUBLIC
My commission exp. Oct. 24, 1997

<u>AGREEMENT</u>

THIS AGREEMENT effective this _10th_ day of _Nov. 1988,_
1988,

BETWEEN:

> DR. CHARLES BRUSCH, M.D., and ~~BRUSCH MEDICAL CENTRE~~, of Cambridge, _15 GROZIER RD. EA._
> Massachusetts, United States of America _02138_
>
> (hereinafter called "Brusch")

OF THE FIRST PART

AND:

> _577 W. 60th Ave. EA._
> ELAINE E. ALEXANDER, of ~~120 West 11th~~
> Avenue, in the City of Vancouver, in the
> Province of British Columbia, Canada, ~~V5V 2V4~~ _V6P1Z8_
>
> (hereinafter called "Alexander")

OF THE SECOND PART

WHEREAS Brusch has formulations for nutritional health supplements and desires to have these products manufactured and distributed worldwide.

AND WHEREAS Alexander has production, marketing, distribution and promotion ability and contacts and is desirous of manufacturing and marketing the Brusch formula products worldwide.

NOW THEREFORE, in consideration of the mutual covenants and conditions hereinafter set forth, the parties hereby covenant and agree as follows:

1.   For the purposes of this agreement the following terms shall have the indicated meanings:

    (a)   "Territory" - the entire world;

(b) "Formula" - any formula for health or nutritional products including, but not limited to, formulations of and based on Rene Caisse's health supplement product;

(c) "Product" - any health or nutritional product or formula over which Brusch has formulation control including, but not limited to, any specialty nutritional, herbal, oil or vitamin product or formula which Brusch obtains;

(d) "Market" - any channel chosen by Alexander to distribute and sell Product in the Territory including, but not limited to:

    (i) multi-level marketing;

    (ii) established distributors to third party retail outlets ("conventional");

    (iii) institutional;

    (iv) mail Order;

    (v) telemarketing;

(e) "Licensed Patent" means any patent for Product owned directly or indirectly by Brusch and such other patents as may be hereafter added hereto by mutual consent of the parties;

(f) "Know-How" means information which is proprietary to Brusch which relates to the manufacture, sale or use of Licensed Product or components thereof and shall include information pertaining to raw materials,

15.   This Agreement shall be governed by and construed in accordance with the Laws of the Province of British Columbia, Canada.

IN WITNESS WHEREOF, Brusch and Alexander have hereunto set their hands and seals on the date first above mentioned

SIGNED, SEALED AND DELIVERED
by **DR. CHARLES BRUSCH** in the
presence of:)
)
_____   )
Witness *Thomas J. Yared*   )   *Dr. Charles Brusch*
)
_____   )   ●
Address *26 STRATFORD ST.*   )   _____
WEST ROXBURY, MA 02132   )   DR. CHARLES BRUSCH
Cambridge - MA. 02138   )
PRINTER   )
Artist-at-home   )
Occupation   )

SIGNED, SEALED AND DELIVERED
by **ELAINE E. ALEXANDER** in the
presence of:)
)
_____   )
Witness *V. Barbon.*   )
)
473-650 W. 41st Ave   )   *Elaine E. Alexander*
_____   )   _____ ●
Address   )   ELAINE E. ALEXANDER
Vancouver, B.C. V5Z 2M9   )
)
TRUST Co. Manager.   )
_____   )
Occupation   )

1348g

TESTIMONIALS

**(Examples of Certified Testimonials regularly
received at Flora Manufacturing and Distributing, Ltd.)**

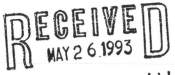

MAY 31,1993
G. SEARS
BOX 125 SITE 6
HYTHE, ALBERTA
TOH 2C0

DEAR SIRS;
     This letter is to thank you and your staff for the help I
recieved from you in obtaining Elaine Alexanders herbal tea
you call "FLOR-ESSENCE".

     I am sure we have all, at one time or another heard of so
called "miracle cures" for one thing and onother, and we have
all been sceptical. This letter is to inform you of me
experience with your product, and how it is making a believer
out of me.

     About 2 years ago my father,(then 84 years old) was
diagnosed with lung cancer and had an operation to remove 2/3
of his right lung. The operation was considered successful and
they "got it all ". About 1 yeas later,(January 1992) Dad was
in California for the winter when he had some very bad back
pains which he thought was the result of a lawn bowling
strain. The pain persisted and on further examination, he was
found to have bone cancer in his spine.On finding this out,
and with medical expences being what they are in the U.S.A.
Dad moved back to Saskatoon where doctors gave him a couple of
radiation treatments which they said had temporarily stopped
the growth but they could do no more. Some time ,I think it
was in Feb. or March, while dad was getting up from a sitting
position he experienced a terrible pain in his back and was
rushed to hospital by ambulance where doctors said a piece of
the growth on his spine had chipped off, and outside of pain
killers there was nothing they could do, and that if it
happened again it could possibly leave him paralysed.This
statement devastated my dad and he was in a very deprassed
state when he visited us in hythe last summer for the wedding
of my son.

     I read an article in Feb. which interested me very much,
the article was about Rene Caisse and her sucesses treating
cancer patients. A friend of mine later claimed he had found
where to obtain some of this tea so I bought some and sent it
to dad. Later my friend phoned Elaine Alexander to see if the
tea he had got for me was in fact esslac. Elaine told him it
was not, but what impressed me the most, was that she didn't
knock it but rather said it may well be just as good as her
tea as she felt it wouldn't be that hard to analyse and
duplicate her tea, she also informed us to get ahold of your
people if we wanted her tea.

     I contacted you and ordered your flor-essence, and sent
some to my dad. In April this year my dad and his wife again
went to California, which supprised me, and a few weeks later
my younger brother, who lives in Saskatoon, called me just to
chat and I learned that before dad left for California,my

brother had taken him to 2 different doctors for a check up and they could find no sign of the cancer.BY the way Dad plans to be up to visit us in June which is a trip I never thought I'd see him make again.

There's more too. I gathered all the information I could find on Rene Caisse and in reading one of the articles where a doctor had taken a terminally ill cancer patient, who also had diabetes,to her and she not only overcame the cancer but also the diabetes. I took that article to a friend of mine in Grande Prairie who had contracted diabeted some 2 years previously and he immediately went to the healthg food store in the mall and bought some. About 3 weeks later he informed me that he had gone from 40 units a day down to 28 units. I must admit, this doesn't mean much to me as I don't know what a unit is, but it sounded like we were on the right track. A couple of weeks later I was attending a meeting that my friend was also at and he said "this is the eighth day I haven't taken any insulin" and said he had gone for a check-up and his doctor said he had only ever heard of this once before and couldn't explain it. I asked my friend if he had told the doctor about drinking the Flor-essence and he said " no he wouldn't believe me anyway" To date he is just over 7 weeks off his insulin. Since talking to you on the phone I found out that my friend had recommended your Flor-essence to another diabetic friend who after three weeks was starting to have a reaction from his insulin shots. I will keep you posted on this case and many others I have since given or recommended your Flor-essence to.

Thanks once again for all your help and a wonderful product.

signed," a believer"
Gordon Sears

Stoneham House Holdings Ltd
Ms. Elaine Alexander (President)
Distributor of "Flor-Essence".

November 12, 1992
William Gaspard
2814 Salmo Court
Vancouver, B.C.
V6T 1N7

Dear Ms. Alexander:

I am writing in regards to the "Flor-Essence" herbal product and how it has turned my mother's health around.

On November 1991 my mother (Elsie Gaspard) was diagnosed with cancer of the throat and stomach and given three months to live. On Boxing Day, my sister Vi heard about your herbal tea (Flor-Essence) from her friend. She purchased some from you, brewed it up and made it available to Mom through the rest of the family. Mom was in bad shape; the doctor said she was too far gone for chemotherapy and prescribed morphine for the pain. He said, just try to keep her comfortable, that was all that can be done. Nobody was very enthusiastic about the herb tea, therefore, she didn't receive it on a regular basis, and she threw up much of that. She was thin as a rail and her eyes were dark sunken circles. She seemed oblivious of everything.

On May 16, an article on "Flor-Essence" came out in the Vancouver Sun. There were several encouraging accounts on how the medicine had amazing results with other cancer patients. Our family became greatly enthusiastic about the medicine. My sister Barbara visited Mom for a while to see that she took the tea on a regular basis. As a result, Mom's health improved dramatically through the months. She gained weight; her appetite and mental capabilities came back.

Best of all, her doctor diagnosed her almost cancer free on or about October 1st, 1992.

Thank you, sincerely

William Gaspard

William Gaspard.

Elsie Gaspard
Ponderosa Lodge
425 Columbia St
Kamloops, BC V5Z 1M9

July 1, 1993
382 Oshawa Blvd. S.
Oshawa, Ontario
L1H 5S5

Elaine Alexander
Flora Distributors Ltd.
7400 Fraser Park Drive
Burnaby B.C.
V5J 5B9

Dear Elaine,

I'm writing to you to thank you for returning my phone call and sending the package with all the information on Flor•Essence® (the improved Essiac formula). Sorry it took so long but there are so many people who needed this information. I have been lending out and photocopying it for others to read. Among the people I shared this information with was a doctor whose little girl had a brain tumour. It was discovered when she suddenly went into a coma. She survived when they shrunk it with radiation, but this was only a temporary measure. They were looking for a solution to get rid of it before it started up again. I hope they consider using Flor•Essence®. It certainly helped me.

When I survived cancer without radiation or chemotherapy the word spread and I was getting calls from people I never met before wondering how this could be. I was shocked at how many people have, or have had cancer. There seems to be an epidemic. It's so bad in this area, that it has been proposed that a hospital that specializes in cancer be built here. It's not surprising when you consider that this is a highly industrialized area.

I also did a lot of reading on the causes of causes cancer and various natural remedies. Find enclosed an interesting article on 714X that I copied for you. I showed it to my doctor, but she says anything injected into the lymph nodes is not a good idea. It can cause disease or infection in this delicate area. She said that if there was a safer way to administer it (orally or injected in the vein or muscle) it might be worth considering. She said that this is not something that I should be thinking about unless the cancer returns and threatens my life. She says that I have bought some time with the surgery – that medical science is moving rapidly at this time and there may be something better if and when I need it.

I certainly agree with her. Just recently I read in the paper about a major breakthrough that is so outstanding we may see people in the near future being treated for and inoculated against this dreaded disease with a safe remedy. If this works out, gone will be the horrors of radiation and chemotherapy.

I should tell you what happened to me. I had a large liposarcoma attached to my kidney. Doctors said it was between the size of a football and a basketball. It was on the right side and pushed all the organs in my abdominal cavity to the left. I looked pregnant and could not sleep on my side because the weight of the tumour would crush my organs and cause great

discomfort.The tumour was pressing against nerves, causing great pain in my right leg and making it too painful to walk. My liver was pushed up into my rib cage causing a great deal of discomfort. I won't go into how this got so big and out-of-hand. It's a long story, but I will tell you how I survived with only surgery.

Because this is a rare form of cancer and it was so far advanced, it was decided by a surgeon in Oshawa to send me to Toronto for an experimental procedure.They would use radiation prior to surgery to shrink the tumour and make it more manageable. It was hoped that this method would make it less likely to return (statistics show 80% chance of recurrence within three years). Nothing could be done after surgery because the organs would cave in, making it hard to aim the radiation in the right area. Chemotherapy was out of the question. It was a one shot deal. If I had radiation this time I could never have it again.

I decided against this procedure because it came with no guarantees, there was not enough evidence over a long enough period of time to convince me it worked, I was afraid that if it did work the radiation would cause another type of cancer, and last but not least I was afraid that nearby vital organs would be damaged. I could not afford any damage to my remaining healthy kidney and I did not want any damage to anything else (stomach, liver, intestines – all these were at risk). I was told the total combined risk was 7%. When you consider what was involved and that it would be weeks before the treatment could start and months before surgery, the only thing I would accept was no risk at all. I said that I would rather live three years with a healthy body than 10 years in misery on dialysis, not to mention further surgery to remove anything else that got damaged by the radiation.

As it turned out I made the right decision. First of all, when I told my brother of the shape I was in he told me about Flor•Essence® and I stated taking it right away. Within days the pain went completely from my leg and I was able to walk. I was eating and sleeping better; even feeling better. The surgery took half the time I was told it would (3hours instead of 6-8). I went into surgery weighing 120lb. and came out weighing 105lb. I was told that he tumour was encased in a hard shell attached to my kidney with a thin thread. They took the kidney and the tumour out and said so far as could be seen they got it all. The odds of it coming back were reduced from 80% to 50%. The incision was a foot long and they used rib stretchers to get at the cancer, so my back was sore for a couple of months. I was off the pain killers permanently 5 days after surgery and was home in a week. Though I tire easily, my recovery has been remarkable. This is partly because I have been seeing a wonderful naturopath.I told her I have been taking your remedy. She has heard of it and says it's a wonderful cleanser.

It looks like the Flor•Essence®. did what the radiation was supposed to do – shrink the tumour and make it behave better for surgery. The only evidence I have to support this is that the pain went from my leg, meaning that something happened to reduce the pressure. I was eating and sleeping better and had a lot more energy.

My naturopath is trying to help me cleanse my body and build up my immune system with natural remedies. Five years ago I spent over 22 years working in a factory with gules and other pollutants. She thinks that this is what weakened my immune system to the point I got cancer and it will take a couple of years of cleansing to get me straightened out. I won't go into the list of vitamins and remedies I take, but I will say that she has a high regard for Flor•Essence® and told me to carry on taking it as part of my cleansing program.

I would like to ask you a few questions about Flor•Essence® because you are the one who has the most knowledge about it. Enclosed find a self-addressed-stamped envelope for your reply.

1. How long should I take Flor•Essence®? My surgery was February 10th and I still take it every day. Is there some point at which it would be safe to stop?

2. What should my present dosage be – the same as before surgery or reduced?

3. Do you think my continued use of Flor•Essence® has destroyed any remaining microscopic cells that would develop into another tumour? Are they gone for good?

4. The articles you sent me say the best method is intramuscular injection of one of the herbs and a tea made our of the balance. If the tumour does come back, is this better than the straight tea? If so, where can I have this done? If the place is too far can my doctor, naturopath or I inject the remedy? If so who would supply it (enclose name, phone number and mailing address) and approximately how much would it cost?

I will not only use this information for myself, but will pass it on to others. Thanks again for your call and all the information. Thanks in advance for your reply to this letter.

Your truly,

Gayle Sutherland

7898 - 118A St.,
Delta, B.C.

Feb. 15, 1993

Flora Distributors,
7400 Fraser Park Drive,
Burnaby, B.C.   V5J 5B9

Dear Sirs:

As a result of breast cancer, I had a partial mastectomy (lumpec-
tomy) in May 1991, followed by five weeks of radiation.

During the year following I did not feel well, lacked energy, and
had numerous health problems (bursitis, severe arthritis pains
in my arms, insomnia, hemorrhoids, etc.)

I started taking Flor-Essence twice a day July 1992. At the end
of the first week my insomnia started to improve noticeably, and
I began to feel well. There have been no signs of arthritis since
I started Flor-Essence, even though I have had mild arthritis pains
in my hands and wrists every fall for years. I also have diverti-
culosis (outpouchings in the weakened walls of the colon) which
causes alternating periods of constipation and diarrhea, and
Flor-Essence has helped this condition to such an extent that my
bowels now feel normal. An added benefit as a result of this is
that the hemorrhoids seem to have disappeared.

Flor-Essence also has a calming effect, and I no longer feel the
need to meditate to relieve stress.

                              Yours truly,

                              P. Campbell
                              Phyllis Campbell

R.J. "Rex" Dawe
2636 Avebury Avenue
Victoria, B.C.
V8R 3W2
(604)595-1637

Jūly 16, 1993

Dear Elaine Alexander:

Am very happy to report that the Prostate/Urinary cleansing herbs you sent me back in february were forwarded to my friend in Ontario and he is greatly improved. In fact, its safe to say he is cured.

Seldom has to get up in the night, no bodily function inconvenience and is back to work. He followed his doctors instructions regarding chemotherapy but cut the 'dosage' in half.

Now he is off chemotherapy completely and is taking the regular Flor-Essence. So chalk up another victory for natural healing Flor-Essence.

By the way, how is the 80 pages cut down to around 40 pages coming along? Catherine and I would be happy to receive a copy when it's convenient.

With best wishes.

Sincerely,

Rex Dawe

July 14, 1993

Mrs. Elaine Alexander,
6690 Oak Street,
Vancouver, B.C.
V6P 3Z2

Dear Mrs. Alexander:

I began taking Florescence in Oct. 1992 to see if it would help my asthma. Even though I had erred in my dosage and was only taking 1 oz. a day, I haven't suffered with my asthma since I began taking it and haven't had to use my Ventolin at all. It is so wonderful, not to have to worry about asthma attacks! Either extreme cold or hot weather would make my asthma flare up, consequently I was always tired and had very sore lungs.

I have also noticed another change and attribute the improvement to Florescence. Over a period of the past 2-3 years, my "creaking bones" were steadily getting worse. When I got out of bed each morning the bones in my feet would sound as though they were all crunching together as I stood on them, my knees would make a horrible,sharp cracking sound each time I bent down, and my joints were constantly stiffening up in my fingers and elbows. I never did see my doctor about it and so I was never diagnosed with having artheritis or osteoporis, but what I do know is that my bones no longer crack. creak, or stiffen up and since my diet and exercise routines haven't changed at all, I contribute the improvement to Florescence!

I am now on the correct dosage of 2 oz. of Florescence a day and look forward to taking Florescence for many years to come! I feel fantastic and have recommended it to quite a few of my friends, with and without illness.

I look forward to receiving your News Letter and attending future seminars. Keep up the good work, you are truly devoted to helping others.

Sincerely,

Sharon Sorensen

Sharon Sorensen,
9089 Draper St.
RR 5
Mission, B.C.
V2V 5X4

Almonte Ont. Nov 27, 1993

Elaine Alexander.

Dear Elaine,

I am writing to you as so many others have done, to let you know of my success in using Flor-Essence. About one year ago I noticed a lump, (on my neck) not larger in diameter than a nickel, and not very high, but growing. Doctors found other smaller lumps on my neck and on Feb 25, 1993 I was told I had rare low grade lymphoma. My family doctor told us that I should immediately start taking Flor-Essence which I did. That same evening.

We talked that week to a man we knew who had, by that time, almost completely cured himself of prostate cancer. He had been examined by the doctors in the cancer clinic and sent home to die.

By March 31st 1993, the date of my first chemotherapy treatment, and even 2 weeks earlier, the lumps on my neck had receded to half the size of Feb 25th.

I took therapy until Aug 24, 1993 when I was told no sign of cancer remained. Clinic doctors seemed surprised that my blood stayed up so well, I had very little side effects from therapy and mostly felt and looked well, through treatment.

I have told many people of Flor-Essence & haug given them literature on its history and what you, Elaine Alexander, have done to promote its use.

My wife and I enjoyed seeing you in Ottawa recently.

I AM ABLE TO HAVE A VERY POSITIVE OUTLOOK FOR THE FUTURE SINCE I FEEL FLOR-ESSENCE IS MY INSURANCE POLICY TO A MUCH LONGER LIFE THAN THE CLINIC DOCTOR PREDICTS. I TAKE IT FAITHFULLY AND WILL NEVER STOP.

I HOPE THAT MANY MANY MORE CANCER PATIENTS AND OTHERS TOO WILL LEARN OF THIS REMEDY OR SHOULD I SAY PREVENTATIVE (BOTH I GUESS) AND HAVE SUCCESS WITH IT.

BEST WISHES TO YOU FOR A CONTINUED HEALTHY HAPPY LIFE + MANY THANKS FOR YOUR GREAT WORK AND HELP.

SINCERELY

Alan Pretty.
Almonte, Ontario, Can.

BOX 861 - 196 GORE ST.

Sep 11/93

Dear Elaine,

My husband was diagnosed
with Prostate Cancer in March of this year.
The Cancer had spead to the lymph node.
We were very concerned. Our son found out
about your herbal tea, and talked us into
going to one of your seminars.

After hearing about all the
positive results that many people had
experienced using FLOR-ESSENCE herbal tea,
my husband reluctantly tried it. He is now
on the Prostate blend as well.

My husband was experiencing
fatigue and tiredness on the combination
hormonal therapy as well as many fregment
trips to the washroom in the middle of
the night.

Presently his PSA is down to
0.2 which is exactly where he should be
even without one of the two hormonal Drugs.
Nighttime trips to the washroom have now
gone to normal

Our whole family believes in
your herbal tea and feel very strong it
has contributed to the excellent results to
date.

We will certenly keep in touch
and thank you for all your sincere help.

With the Testosterone of 0.3 we made love, the

Dr. thought it was funny, and we think it is wonderful.

Thank you so much

Yours Truly

Elfriede Hom

Mr and Mrs. A. Hari
12318 - 56th Ave.
Surrey, B.C.
V3X 2X2

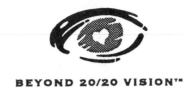

October 15, 1993

RECEIVED
OCT 21 1993
Flora Distributors Ltd.

Flora Manufacturing & Dist. Ltd.
7400 Fraser Park Drive
Burnaby, B.C. V5J 5B9

Dear Sirs/Madam:

I am really excited to be writing to you at this time to share my story of success using the Flor-Essence distributed by your company. I understand that as a thank you for my sharing you will provide me with some complimentary Flor-Essence product and look forward to receiving that. Please feel free to use my personal experience or excerpts of it in order that more people are informed and encouraged to used natural products to help themselves.

My Amazing Experience with Flor-Essence

I became pregnant in early April of 1993 and by early July, I had a discharge of what appeared initially to be a part of the endometrium. One month later it was discovered that I had actually had a miscarriage and the specialist I was seeing sent me for an ultrasound. Sure enough there was some mass in my uterus and a surgical procedure called D&C was recommended. Now, just one year earlier I had also become pregnant and discovered that I had a mole instead of a fetus growing inside of me and I did in fact go through with the D&C procedure. It was quite unpleasant to have to deal with my body's reaction to the injection of antibiotics and the anaesthesia for the surgery. It put me out of commission for almost a full week. I did not want to repeat this invasive surgical procedure and began to explore natural methods for eliminating the mass. I started on a regime of herbal tinctures which were to help tone the whole uterus and help move through what was inside. After some time, I realized that I needed something stronger than what I was taking and a friend suggested that I try Flor-Essence as she had cured her overian cysts that way.

I began taking Flor-Essence in mid-September and, after only two days on it, I started discharging lumps of material and was bleeding like I was having a menstrual period. However, it was quite heavy with thick discharge mixed in with lumps or clots of old blood. After one week on Flor-Essence I went for another ultrasound and was informed that the mass inside the uterus was thinner and appeared to moving downward towards the cervix. Encouraged by these results I continued with the daily dosage of Flor-Essence and after the 2nd week of taking it I started to experience really strong and rather painful cramps (felt almost like I was birthing) during the mid-day for 2-3 hours at a time. I knew something big was happening and decided to just get into the pain and eased it by putting a heating pad on my tummy and relaxing into it. After three or four days of

these intense cramps I went to the washroom and out slipped a mass of old birth material which was roughly the size of a tampon. Immediately after discharging this piece of material the bleeding subsided and by the next day I was no longer bleeding. Deep inside I was convinced that everything was now cleared up and thought that another ultrasound was in order to confirm this.   We were in the process of moving out of the city when all of this was happening, so after having had a chance to settle in a bit I arranged to have a third ultrasound and have heard just today, October 15, 1993 that my uterus is now back to normal and nothing further needs to be done. Can't tell you how relieved and thankful I am for Flor-Essence.

Thank you again for your support in my sharing this experience with you.

Very sincerely yours,

Lise Kaplan
Executive Director

9

Mr. & Mrs. Jack Dzoeshout
7149 Douglas Cr.
Niagara Falls, Ont. L2G 3C3

Niagara Falls July 26/93.

Dear Elaine Alexander.

First of all I thank for the Phone call and conversation about the herbs I bought some and made my own tea it work out fine I have taken it now since I talk to you also my doctor told me to go ahead and take it I have the operation done on July 9-93 but to my suprise I had two operation done they removed my prostate and found that my artery in my leg was block up so one other specilist performed a second operation a bypas in the groun of my leg so the recovery was harder but everthing is fine now. When I came home from the hospital I went back on the tea and believe me I feel much better I met 3 peaple with the same problem and told them about you I know that one lady talk to you about her mother and yesterday I talk to the lady she told me that her mother is on the Tea and feels better I hope that I can help some more people and that the good Lord my bless you for as long you live I also recieved the booklet and made some copies of it to give to people to read those remarceble stories Now dear Elaine I close this letter with the beste thanks out of the bottom of my heart and I hope that the Good Lord bless you for all the work you have done

your truly Jack Dzoeshout

4603- Bowness Rd. N.W.
Calgary Alberta.
T3B 0B2.

Aug 10 - 93

Dear Elaine,

We wanted you to know, that since Ed found out he had prostate cancer in Oct. 92 he has been taking Flor-Essence & Elypis herbal drink.

Ed could not have his cancerous prostate removed, because of his weakened heart condition. He did have a biopsy operation, that showed the cancer was just starting to spread. He then had 37 treatments of Radiation over a 2 month period. Ed suffered from bladder & bowel irritations throughout. But he feels that due to his taking the Flor-Essence & Elypis herbal drinks he was spared from further side effects.

Ed also feels, that had he not had the benifits of the herbal drinks, he would not be so well today.

He had an M.R.1. Scan, & the results come back that he is 100% cancer free. He has decided to continue to use the herbal drinks for the rest of his life.

We are so grateful that I saw your article in the Calgary Herald.

Sincerely

Ed Florkow   and

Hannah Florkow.

Henry P. Wilder
417 Monarch Bay
Dana Point, Ca. 92629

August 31, 1993

Dear Elaine,

It was so nice to talk with you yesterday. And I want to thank you again for shipping the special prostate cancer package. I really think I should pay something for it. At least I will send you the postage and hope you won't mind.

When I gave the order to Susan Martin she said she didn't have the special prostate package yet, but that she would contact you and have you send it.

I have been taking the Flor-Essence only for about a five week period. In that time my PSA dropped from 322.0 to 286.5. This is a tremendous drop and I'm very confident that it will continue to go down. I have had no side effects from the added dosage. Normally I have been taking the other tea twice a day, in the morning before breakfast and at night when I go to bed. I'm now taking the Flor-Essence plus the special prostate package three times per day. The second dose is in the middle of the afternoon.

I have just come from my Doctor's office and he thinks this is terrific and wanted information about the product and the address of Flora Inc. in Lynden, Wa.

Keep up the good work and we hope everything is going well with you.

Cordially, Henry

CC Susan Martin

Woodbridge - Ontario. L4L 7V1   Thursday, April 22
62 BLAINE COURT   199

Dear Ms. Alexander,

Thank you very much for your
earnest concern about my father's condition. I would
like to let you know how impressed and overwhelmed
I am, for your honest interest, also how happy I am
I was able to talk to you at the seminar in Toron'

As I've already told you, my father was diagno
with adeno-carcinoma on the prostate gland in Oct. 9
Please, look at the enclosed copy of the doctor's diagno
The therapy suggested, was radiotherapy without chen
However, due to personal reasons, my father had to
leave for Cyprus in November 92' upon which time
I gave him 2 bottles of the liquid Flor. Essence whic
he was taking morning and evening, 2 ounces at eac
time as per instructions. In February /93, he went
to a specialist in Cyprus to be re-examined and
assess the possibility of having the radiotherapy
there, instead of coming back to Canada.

The initial examination showed no cancer. I contact
the doctor in Cyprus and asked him to perform the same
biopsy my father had done in Toronto, i.e. transrecto
biopsy. The enclosed copy of the results speaks for
itself. No evidence of cancer, only the Cypriot doctor
suggests a hormone therapy just because the Canadia
biopsy showed adeno-ca. We were overwhelmed,
surprised at the fast results! I still can't believe
Flor. Essence worked so fast on my father, who, by

the way, is not a very good keeper of diet or health regiments. He consumes a lot of sugar (which as you said to me, in Toronto, is an enemy for cancer patients!)

I sent him more supplies of Flor-Essence and told him to continue taking it, but my real triumph will be when I convince him to come back to Toronto to be checked again by the same doctor who originally found the cancer!

I have an appointment to talk to my doctor and tell him about the turnaround of my father's condition but I really don't think he will attribute it to Flor-Essence. We discussed it before and he doesn't believe in herbal remedies. I'm anxious to see, though, how he is going to explain the sudden disappearance of cancer in 2 months.

Enclosed are all the facts of my father's condition, before and after the Flor-Essence.

I have 2 more friends, one in Windsor, Ontario, the other one in Hamilton who have both lymphatic cancer and are taking Flor-Essence. The first lady in Windsor is also under another experimental treatment. If you would like to talk to her, please let me know, I will give her name and phone no. She needs all the support and encouragement!

In our circle of friends, I was perhaps, the first one to know about Essiac back in 1977, from Homemakers magaz. I'm so sad that the government has not even allowed it as a mercy remedy for those who have no other hope! They have other drugs which are supplied on mercy grounds for Aids and other incurable diseases!

Do you think that ~~Essiac~~ Flor-Essence will be ever allowed to prove its miraculous effect on cancer patients? How can we, ~~the people~~ who know Flor Essence ~~Essiac~~ help to make it known to those who need it?

Please, acknowledge receipt of my letter.
Promising to keep in touch! Regards
Elli Eleftheriou.

YORK-FINCH GENERAL HOSPITAL

OPERATIVE REPORT   (PRIVATE AND CONFIDENTIAL)

UNIT NO: 180578   ROOM:

NAME: PETRIDES, PETROS`   DOCTOR: ████████

AGE: ADMITTED:

DATE OF OPERATION: 2/10/92   cc: Dr. S. Salkauskis

PRE-OPERATIVE DIAGNOSIS: Bladder irrigation and prostatic nodule.

POST-OPERATIVE DIAGNOSIS: Same.

OPERATION: Cystoscopy and needle biopsy of the prostate gland.

SURGEON: Dr. Kong.   ASSISTANT:

ANAESTHETIST:

ANAESTHETIC: Local.

CLINICAL NOTE:

This elderly gentleman has had a long history of bladder irritation with frequent
nocturia and urinary frequency, as well as suprapubic pressure and post-void dribbling.
He had TURP in 1989 and further examination never demonstrated any significant
obstructive lesion.

On this occasion, he was found to have PSA up to 15, along with a small palpable
nodule at the apex. Therefore, biopsy was to be carried out, along with a cystoscopy.

OPERATIVE PROCEDURE:

The patient was prepped and draped in the semi-lithotomy position. Panendoscopy
demonstrated a normal anterior urethra. There was no stricture and the prostate was
wide open. The prostate was non-obstructive. The bladder neck, however, scarred down
and was slightly stenotic. There was no significant post-void residual volume in the
bladder and the bladder was free of trabeculation, tumor or stone. The instrument was
withdrawn. Bimanual examination again demonstrated a 5 mm nodule at the apex of the
prostate which appears to be scar from previous operation. Biopsies were taken
transrectally.

The patient tolerated the procedure well and is to be followed in the office in a
week's time.

YPK/pf   Y. P. KONG, M.D.

Dictated: 2/10/92
Processed: 6/10/92

YORK-FINCH GENERAL HOSPITAL

DEPT OF NUCLEAR MEDICINE (PRIVATE & CONFIDENTIAL)

UNIT NO: ROOM: OP

NAME: PETROS, PETRIDES   DOCTOR: Kong/Salkauskis

AGE: 76   DISCHARGED:

DATE OF INVESTIGATION 21 Oct 92

---

24 HR. RADIOIODINE UPTAKE (N = 7 - 30%)
(LOW VALUES DO NOT NECESSARILY INDICATE
HYPOTHYROIDISM)

NAME OF SCAN: TOTAL BODY BONE SCAN

ISOTOPE: 99 mTc methylene diphosphate

DOSE: 552 MBq

INTERPRETATION:

A scan of the skull, axial skeleton, ribs, shoulders, pelvis and hips was done.

The uptake and distribution of radionuclide throughout the bony structures
visualized appears normal.

H. COOPERSMITH, M.D.

HC/pf
Dictated: 22.10.92
Processed: 22.10.92

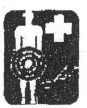

ΟΥΡΟΛΟΓΙΚΟ ΚΕΝΤΡΟ ΥΨΗΛΗΣ ΤΕΧΝΟΛΟΓΙΑΣ ΕΥΑΓΓΕΛΙΣΤΡΙΑ ΑΤΛ | **UROLOGICAL CENTER OF HIGH TECHNOLOGY EVANGELISTRIA LTD**

Dr. ACHILLEAS G. KORELLIS, M.D.	Δρ. ΑΧΙΛΛΕΑΣ Γ. ΚΟΡΕΛΛΗΣ, Μ.D=
SPECIALIST UROLOGIST SURGEON	ΞΙΔΙΚΟΣ ΧΕΙΡΟΥΡΓΟΣ ΟΥΡΟΛΟΓΟΣ
Bremen West Germany	Βρέμης Δυτικής Γερμανίας
1 GEORGALLA, NICOSIA 162	ΠΩΡΓΑΛΛΑ 1, ΛΕΥΚΩΣΙΑ 162
TEL. 368546, 441580 FAX 417383	ΤΗΛ. 868546, 441580, ΦΑΞ 46736

MEDICAL REPORT 5/4/93

RE: PETROS PETRIDES

The above named patient came to see me on the 18th/1/93, complaining of urgency and nocturnia. His medical history especially from urological aspect was a TURP in the year 198 in Canada and a prostate biopsy 10/92. The ultrasound of the urinary bladder evaluated residual urine of 60ml. The urethrocystoscopy was normal without evidence of prostate ca. On the 18th/3/93 a transrektal biopsy was done. It shows predominantly necrotic hyalinized degenerated tissue. No evidence of

x no-Ca. Because of the biopsy results in Canada -10/92- which showed adeno-ca I suggest antiandrogen-therapy i.typ. f. also an depot 300 mg i. m. once a month

UROLOGICAL CENTRE
OF HIGH TECHNOLOGY
EVANGELISTRIA LTD

Dr. ΑΧΙΛΛΕΑΣ ΚΟΡΕΛΛΗΣ
ΧΕΙΡ. ΟΥΡΟΛΟΓΟΣ

NICOSIA - CYPRUS.

(NICOSIA - CYPRUS)

NAME: PETRIDES, PETROS

DOB/AGE: 18/6/16   DIS.DATE:

SURGEON: Kong ✓

DOCTOR: Salkauskis

YORK - FINCH GENERAL HOSPITAL

SURGICAL PATHOLOGY REPORT

SPECIMEN NO: S-6749-92

MATERIAL   Biopsy of prostate

CLINICAL DIAGNOSIS

DATE RECEIVED ___Oct 02/92___

GROSS DESCRIPTION:

Specimen received consists of two elongated length of greyish-tan soft tissue. They vary in diameter from less than 0.1 at end to 0.1 cm at the other. They range in length from approximately 1.6 to 2 cm. Specimen is totally submitted in one block.

BO/vj
Dictated: 02/10/92
Processed: 05/10/92

DIAGNOSIS:

Adenocarcinoma and biopsy of prostate gland.

Code 4.

B. OLIVER, M.D.

BO:vj
Dictated: 05/10/92
Processed: 05/10/92

august 02 nd 1993

Mrs. Elaine Alexander
C/o FLORA Ltd
7400 Fraser Park Drive
Burnaby, BC
V5J 5B9

Dear Mrs. Alexander

My wife Lisette and I, were so happy to meet you at your conference of may 1993 in Ste-Foy (Quebec).

As we talked together concerning the success of FLORESSENCE in my case, please find enclosed a summary of my medical record to testity this success.

Now I can say, the hope is in FLORESSENCE, because since 1987, it's the first time, I can walk without a cane, no more medication, with the shape of my twenty age(42).

I'm sorry to send this only in french, I'm not verry good in translation, but I know FLORA got a translator at lease Jim Stott got Pierre Lefracois in Montreal. If you need more information's or any collaboration contact me, I'm available any time.

Enjoyment to meet you again, yours truly,

Gilles Rioux

One morning, when I woke up in the spring of 1974, I realized that both of my legs were quite heavy and that I could no longer move them. Gradually after a week's time, I was able to move them slightly. I was hospitalized for a few weeks. When I finally got out, I had to walk with a cane for many months. In the fall of 1980 I began having blood pressure problems which I was able to control with the help of medication. Following surgery for the removal of a slipped disc in the spring of 1986, problems with my equilibrium, with dizziness, with unexplained fatigue and with my vision appeared. I began having bladder control problems in the beginning of 1987 and in the summer, I became paralyzed once again but only on the left side.

From 1987 to 1992 I paralyzed seven times. Doctors had diagnosed me as having MULTIPLE SCLEROSIS, NEUROGENIC BLADDER, ESSENTIAL LABILE BLOOD PRESSURE. I lived from my bed to my wheelchair, never leaving my cane behind. Only in 1990 was I hospitalized for 154 days, following that incident I had to resign myself to quitting my job. I don't have to mention that mentally I was not doing too well. I was being treated by neurologists, urologists, nephrologists, psychiatrists, physiotherapists and occupational therapists. I took a lot of medication: many of which were steroid and cortisone treatments. I wore a prothesis on my left foot for over one year.

At the end of November 1992, I had heard of Flor.Essence and it was only at the end of January 1993 that I began my treatment. In the beginning I took 3 doses of 56 ml daily which was reduced after two weeks to 2 doses of 56 ml per day. During that same period I followed a rehabilitation program that was offered by a rehabilitation center in my area. After 4 weeks I began to notice that my fatigue had substantially decreased and nonetheless, I found some hidden strengths that had been previously lost.

For the very first time at the end of April 1993, I walked without a cane. I was physically evaluated at the time I had started my rehabilitation program and when I completed the program at the end of May 1993, I had improved by more than 200%.

On this day, August 1st, 1993, I walk without a cane, I no longer take any medication, my physical state is almost back to normal and the problems with my equilibrium, my dizziness, my vision, my fatigue and my bladder have all disappeared. My mental state is quite good. At the age of 42 with a Multiple Sclerosis label, I thank God that I am aware of Flor.Essence, a magic potion that convinces me that my quality of life can improve.

Gilles Rioux

About The Author:

At the relatively young age of 47, Richard Thomas has experienced many interesting and challenging careers. He has worked as a *commercial pilot, english teacher, commodity trader, investment advisor,* and for the past ten years, a highly sought after *copy writer* in the burgeoning field of health and fitness. He has written, produced, and managed numerous successful marketing campaigns, both nationally and internationally.

Recently, due to his own widening spiritual interests he has chosen to dedicate his talents to writing informative *in depth works* about what he considers to be the world's most important and *unknown* natural health discoveries. *The Essiac Report* is his first effort in what he hopes will be a long and fruitful series of work that will help to further enlighten the public about God's miracle of natural healing. Richard Thomas lives with his wife, cat and two dogs, in Los Angeles, California.